$f\mathbf{P}$

"Dr. Phil has cut through the confusion of fad diets with clinically supported sound information and action plans for lasting weight management. *The Ultimate Weight Solution: The 7 Keys to Weight Loss Freedom* introduces a strategy that is based on scientifically sound information about nutrition and physical activity. The American Heart Association recognizes that obesity, a major risk factor for heart disease, is a growing worldwide problem that must be addressed by providing the public with the best information possible. Dr. McGraw's book clearly sets forth a plan for prevention and treatment of obesity."

—Robert. H. Eckel, M.D., Professor of Medicine,
Physiology and Biophysics, University of Colorado Health
Sciences Center; Chair, Council on Nutrition, Physical
Activity and Metabolism, American Heart Association

The Ultimate Weight Solution

The 7 Keys to
Weight Loss Freedom

Dr. Phil McGraw

*f*P

Free Press

New York London Toronto Sydney Singapore

THE FREE PRESS
A Division of Simon & Schuster, Inc.
1230 Avenue of the Americas
New York, NY 10020

THE FREE PRESS and colophon are trademarks
of Simon & Schuster, Inc.

For information regarding special discounts for bulk purchases,
please contact Simon & Schuster Special Sales:
1-800-456-6798 or business@simonandschuster.com

Designed by Nancy Singer

Manufactured in the United States of America

10   9   8   7   6   5   4   3   2   1

Library of Congress Cataloging-in-Publication Data is available.

ISBN 0-7432-3674-2

To Robin, my wife and inseparable companion,
who created for herself and for our family the very kind
of lifestyle this book seeks to inspire;
and to our sons Jay and Jordan,
who are the epitome of health and energy;
and to my mother, "Grandma Jerry," and my
deceased father, Joe, for teaching me to never
settle for less than my dreams.

And especially,

To all of those people who are sick to death of riding the
"diet roller coaster" in pursuit of the elusive goal of a fit and trim life.

Acknowledgments

The Ultimate Weight Solution is the culmination of thirty years of treating, living, learning, and researching the challenges of obesity. It has been a passion-driven project during which I have had the privilege of working with an absolutely incredible team of dedicated and caring people who have worked tirelessly to bring together what I believe is a definitive work on the management of obesity.

Thanks to my wife, Robin, for always living and managing your personal life in such an inspirational manner. (I so married over my head!) You make it an undeniable truth that by embracing self-respect and the choices that naturally flow from it, health, fitness, and graceful progression through life can be fun and exciting rather than dull and self-denying. Regarding your body and mind as a gift to be managed with dignity has made the three boys in your life do a better job by just trying to keep up!

Thanks to our sons Jay and Jordan for always supporting and being proud of your dad and making it easy for me to be proud of you. Your spark and energy keep me young and challenge me to keep reaching for the next level and the next "big thing." And thanks, Jordan, for getting good enough on the electric guitar that it is not painful to listen to you play while I try to write! You guys are what it's all about for ol' dad.

I once again thank my dear friend Oprah for her unwavering commitment to helping me get my messages about human functioning out into the world. Thanks for always being such a passionate supporter and an honest source of feedback in all that I strive to do. Your friendship and kindness are more appreciated than you ever could know. Your belief in and commitment to my success are and have been invaluable. Thanks especially for all of your input after such a careful reading of the manuscript and for coming up with such a great title for the book! Having Oprah for an "editor" ain't a half-bad deal!

A special thanks to G. Frank Lawlis, Ph.D., for his tireless work on this book from the very moment of its conception. Dr. Lawlis is, in my opinion, the greatest psychologist alive today and has been a guiding light to me personally and professionally for almost thirty years now. Frank, your knowledge of psychology in general and the behavioral medicine approaches to the treatment of obesity in particular are encyclopedic and invaluable. Your ability to tie together the many dimensions of the complex human mind and emotions has added much to the clarity I sought in creating a "how-to" manual for the reader. Your creative thinking and the translation of those ideas into words on the page is among your many world-class skills. Thank you, too, for your help in the massive review of more than thirty years of obesity research in the psychological literature. Above all else, thanks for your friendship and caring.

Thanks especially to Maggie Robinson, Ph.D. Dr. Robinson is clearly the preeminent nutritionist in America today, and her tireless work on content, organization, flow, and writing was invaluable. Maggie has made *The Ultimate Weight Solution* a better book in a number of ways. If we could all remember even a fraction of the nutritional science that Maggie added to this book we would have the battle half-won. Thanks, Maggie, for "raising the bar" and always having such a positive and infectiously passionate spirit. You made this project fun and taught me a tremendous amount. You are a great writer and I am proud to call you friend.

Thanks also to Tom Diaz, M.D., for the cutting-edge medical counsel on the content of this book. When I sought a medical consultant on this project, I wanted the absolute best of the best. As I reviewed the many résumés submitted, the choice was clear: there was Dr. Diaz and then there was everybody else. Dr. Diaz is one of those doctors who treat the patient and not just the disorder or disease. In short, Dr. Diaz gets it. Tom, your expertise in obesity, aging, and longevity was invaluable and allowed me to merge the psychological and medical aspects of weight management into a coherent whole. Thanks especially for your review of the massive medical literature on this important subject and for all of your own research specifically done for the book. The hours you put in were countless and the energy never waning. Thanks also for solving the mystery of my personal chemistry; you have undoubtedly added years and years to my life. Thanks for always being there for me and mine.

Thanks also to P.J. Skerrett, editor of Harvard Medical School's highly regarded *Harvard Heart Letter,* for his most thorough and helpful review of the manuscript technically and content wise. P.J., your knowledge of and rapport with the state of the art in obesity management was extremely helpful. Your critique confirmed our direction and content and refined the book in important ways.

Thanks to the American Heart Association (AHA) and Robert H. Eckel, M.D.—Professor of Medicine, Physiology, and Biophysics, University of Colorado Health Sciences Center Denver, and Chairman of the American Heart Association's Council on Nutrition, Physical Activity, and Metabolism—for reviewing and critiquing *The Ultimate Weight Solution.* The AHA committee and Dr. Eckel made this a better book, particularly in the technical areas. The work of the AHA is unrivaled in the quest to raise the awareness of Americans in the area of heart health and the related need for weight control. Being a part of that important undertaking is a privilege.

Thanks to Jan Miller, literary agent extraordinaire, and her entire staff at Dupree Miller and Associates in Dallas, Texas. Jan's number-one priority seems to be making sure that just about everybody in this world reads my books. And I do believe if anyone can achieve such a thing, it is definitely the amazing Jan Miller. Jan, your tireless advocacy and your willingness to charge any "machine-gun nest" to get things done and done right are hugely appreciated. You have an incredibly powerful "secret weapon" in Shannon Miser-Marven. Shannon is one of a kind and is the consummate professional. The fact that you two are so committed to getting things exactly, precisely right, every single time, has made this book appreciably better. Thanks for caring so much about what we do.

Thanks as always to Gary Dobbs, my best friend, partner, and confidant. You are always in my balcony supporting all that I do and caring so much about my family and me. I could not have done this without your support and input from so many different angles. I appreciate your early and ongoing review of this manuscript and your invaluable suggestions to improve it. You are greatly appreciated.

Thanks to Scott Madsen, my friend and associate, for always

doing whatever it takes to get whatever needs doing done. I appreciate your willing spirit and boundless energy, both of which directly created the time to do this project. Thanks also to Dave Khan for all your hard work in keeping things rolling while I worked on this book.

Thanks to Terry Wood, Carla Pennington, Gwynne Thomas, Kandi Amelon, and Angie Kraus, my world-class team of associates that create the *Dr. Phil Show* everyday. Thanks for all of the feedback on the early drafts of the manuscript and for continuing to be my "feminine side."

My appreciation also to Carolyn Reidy, President, Simon & Schuster Adult Publishing Group, and Dominick Anfuso, my in-house editor, for sharing the vision of creating a book designed to stem the tide of obesity in America. And for committing to aggressively getting the book into the hands of those who would read and act upon it.

Contents

Part One

UNLOCKING THE DOORS TO PERMANENT WEIGHT LOSS

1

Getting Real About You and Your Weight

Change can come in either of two important ways:
Start behaving positively or stop behaving negatively.
—DR. PHIL

You have a decision to make.

You know it and so do I. At this very moment, you are standing in the aisle of a bookstore, or at an airport, thumbing through these pages, or you are sitting at home, reading this book. You are thinking about your weight and how you have tried to lose it in a million wrong ways. You are wondering if maybe, just maybe, there is something here for you, something you have wanted for a very long time. And if there is, should you try it?

But hear me out: this decision you are mulling over in your head is not whether to start yet another "diet." You have made that well-intentioned but misguided choice dozens of times. And through it all, your weight just keeps creeping up or maybe even shooting sky-high, and it is getting harder to control with each passing year.

The decision you must make is whether or not you will quit conning yourself and telling yourself what you so desperately wish were the truth: that there is some hot new diet out there, promising quick and easy results. So decide: do you want to keep fooling yourself or not? Do you want to keep chasing after, and being seduced by, "miracle" diets, slimming products, and "overnight" weight loss? You've known for a long time that you were going to have to get real about fat or stay real fat. But if you had done what I'm about to ask you to do, instead of going on that last diet you started or signing up for that last program, this decision would be behind you right now.

Let me be real clear: despite the millions of advertising dollars spent to convince you otherwise, losing weight and keeping it off is not "quick and easy," and you know it. You know as well as I do that what I'm saying is the way it is. You know it because you have been on umpteen diets, from the cabbage soup diet to the water diet, and not one of them has ever kept you slender and fit. You have always known that these quick fixes don't work, but it was fun to believe it, at least at first, until everything you tried brought you back to the same point of failure.

I have to get totally real with you: I know you are looking for something you can take tonight that promises slim tomorrow. I know you're looking for something that melts fat off like the sun melts ice. I know you want these things, but continuing to chase after them will bring you nothing but frustration, pain, and self-remorse. You will just continue to sell yourself short, stay stuck in your life and struggle day after day with overeating and being overweight, never doing anything constructive about it.

But stop right here: if you adopt what I will give you on every page of this book, you will overcome your weight challenges and struggles. Nothing will stop you from being anything other than healthy, vibrant, in shape, and fully in charge of yourself and everything you think, do, and feel. This will happen because you make it happen. It will happen because you have made the decision to step up and do what it takes to have what you want.

As we go through this book together, you will discover that unlike most lose-weight programs out there, there is no "one size fits all" solution (no pun intended!) to responsible and permanent weight control. It just doesn't work that way. Because you are a unique individual, your weight-control issues are unique, as well. The strategies you require must be yours and yours alone. Any plan that creates lasting, for-life results is going to have to be designed specifically for you, by you, with help from someone who has done his homework and has broken the code of what is truly required for you to lose weight and keep it off. That someone is me.

For more than thirty years, I have counseled people just like you, people battling weight problems, ranging from chronic obesity to life-threatening eating disorders, and I understand the impact on their life not just from a professional standpoint, but from a personal one as well. In 1995 my father, who struggled for years with weight-related heart disease, collapsed and died suddenly of a heart attack one Sunday morning while teaching Sunday school at his church. Obesity robbed him of many precious years of his life, and it has gravely affected the health of many other members of my family. To say the least, I am painfully aware of the toll obesity can take on every dimension of your life and health. Over these many years of counseling overweight patients, I have discovered what it takes for you to create the results you want. That means I know how you can get your weight and your life under control and back on the right track, permanently.

When you follow my instructions and take the decisive and effective action I will detail for you, you will begin to live with such a high level of health, energy, vitality, and control that your life will seem like new. And you will never have to revert to your old, overweight self again—ever. Trust me, you are going to get there faster with this approach than if you had followed all the fad diets in the world, one right after the other. Whatever your current weight or diet history, this is something that you can do. All it requires is a willing spirit and an open mind.

I am not one to jump on my own bandwagon, but there was an eight-year period in my career during which my work focused particularly on people who were 100, 200, 300, or more pounds overweight—men and women who would normally be written off as "hopeless cases"—most of them emptied of any expectancy for ever scaling down to a normal weight. The approaches I used with them are precisely the very same get-real strategies for weight loss you will learn about and apply here. That said, I will skip to the end of the story and tell you that, significantly, more than 80 percent of these patients not only lost their excess weight, they kept it off. (Regarding that 80-plus percent success rate, know that these kinds of numbers are amazingly rare and fly in the face of the outcome of conventional diet programs, which, embarrassingly, can claim barely a 5 percent "success" rate. Put another way, this means that dieting has a 95 percent failure rate. Ninety-five percent of all people who lose weight gain it all back, with interest, within a few years. Not very good odds, not good at all. You wouldn't gamble your money if those were the odds, if out of every 100 spins, rolls, or poker hands, you'd lose 95 times. You'd go broke. Same deal here: stop gambling with your weight and your health.)

I'm so confident about what I'm giving you in this book because it is not only from my own professional experience, but it is also from what the most current research into weight control suggests. I reviewed every piece of quality research I could find in the psychological and medical literature. You're going to learn the scientific and proven truth, the reality, and the honest-to-God deal about those things that can genuinely help you when you take action and do your part. It's information that you won't get from the weight loss gurus and the diet industry because it can't be Madison-Avenued into new diet schemes. What I've done for you is to distill all the relevant information you need, from my clinical practice and from the research on who keeps weight off and who doesn't, into a coherent, doable plan that will help you do this right, one time, beginning now. Up until this point, you just haven't had the answers, the knowledge, the tools, the inside scoop you need to initiate and sustain lasting change. Now you do; now you will have what you need. But for you to succeed, you have to translate this knowledge, awareness, and insight into action. I will show you how on every single page of this book. This is not brain surgery, not even close. There is, however, a science to these matters. And I know the science. So if you will do what I am about to set out for you, you will lose your unwanted weight and you will keep it off. If you don't, you won't. It's just that simple. Further, what you are about to do doesn't work some of the time, it works all of the time.

But let me warn you: I'm not going to tell you what you want to hear. I'm going to tell it like it is, even though that may be difficult to hear. I'm going to tell you the truth, and in so doing, stop this ridiculous roller-coaster ride you have been on for way too long. What's more, experience has taught me that effective weight control will never be "quick and easy," but it is doable. The reason no one has ever told you the truth is simply that "quick and easy" sells a whole lot better than "doable!" I promise you that "doable" works because the quickest route from A to Z, from what your weight is now to what you want it to be, is not at some hurry-up, panicked, fevered pace. If you are going to get the results you want, the fastest way is by following the plan I will outline for you here.

Maybe right now, as you read these words, you are all pumped up, emotionally energized, motivated to the max, about getting started. That's fine, but let me caution you: even if you have all of the desire or "want to" in the world, this is not enough if you don't know "what" to do and "how" to do it. Think about it: if all of a sudden you were strapped into the cockpit of a Boeing 777 at 40,000 feet and forced to "land or die," you would be highly, highly motivated to succeed. But no matter how much "want to" you had, you would not get that airplane on the ground in one piece. Without some very specific knowledge of speeds, power settings, and procedures, you would crash. Same deal here!

Maybe, on the other hand, you are completely deflated because of your latest frustrating attempt at weight loss. Maybe you feel demoralized and feel a sting of shame over your size. Maybe your weight problem is draining your life energy day by day, and making you feel miserable about yourself and your future. You've internalized a feeling of powerlessness, and every time you try and fail, you subject yourself to more of the same. If you have lived like this for very long, you may have developed an underlying hopelessness. Well, don't you give in to it! No matter how many diets you've tried, no matter how many times you've failed in the past, no matter if you haven't seen your feet in forty years, I want you to stop selling yourself short and reach in a mature and strategic way for all you are capable of doing, being, and having.

If you are ever to get started on the right path to change, there is one important precondition you have to meet. You must rid yourself of that gnawing and overpowering sense of urgency and panic that always seems to appear on the scene, like ants spoiling the fun at a picnic, every time you decide to lose weight or otherwise get in shape. You know these feelings; they nag at you with words like *you have to be skinny by summer . . . you have to be buffed by your birthday . . . you have to be thin for that job interview . . . you have do this or that,* and so it goes, relentlessly tormenting you to the point of making you want to give up before you start. Go on alert here that this is the language of losers, and if you rely on it, always telling yourself that you have to do something about your plight, you will subvert your own best interests. And the prospect of losing weight and getting healthier will be less agreeable and less manageable with each passing day.

So listen to me: you do not have to do anything. You always have a choice. You can choose to obsess about your weight, or not. You can choose to worry about it, or not. You can choose to panic about your situation, or not. When you choose your behavior and your thoughts, you choose the consequences that flow from those choices. So you must start choosing differently, right here and right now, by being open to this book and everything in it.

Stop telling yourself that you just absolutely "have to" lose weight, because that's a lie. You don't "have to" lose weight. You may want to, you may even need to, but you don't have to. It would be nice if you did, but it isn't something you must do. That's just what you have been telling yourself because you thought it would motivate you. Lying to yourself like this won't help you; trust me. You have to breathe—no choice there—but you don't have to lose weight. So instead of all that drama and self-recrimination, I want you to choose to feel very calm and very relaxed. Get up each morning, look at yourself in the mirror, and see yourself not as someone who is overweight or out of shape, but as the someone you will become, a person with a greater level of dignity and worth who, for probably the first time ever, is finally going to succeed—for a lifetime.

As my friend Maya Angelou has so wisely said, "You did what you knew how to do, and when you knew better, you did better." That's where I want you to be at this point in your life. Whatever you did in the past to try to lose weight, you did what you knew how to do. But as we work together through this book, you will know better and you will do better—a whole lot better!

Trust me, you will succeed—you will do this right, one time—because you are about to take your weight-control efforts to a deeper level, where you exercise your personal power to be totally and consciously in charge of everything you think, do, and feel. It's not just about cutting calories, doing a few more push-ups, or taking diet pills. It's not simply about just getting "skinny." It's about changing what you eat, why you eat, where you eat, when you eat, and how you eat, and doing it all in a way that is custom-designed so that it is natural for *you*. It's about changing yourself from the inside out, so that being what is fit and healthy for you is as natural and as normal as breathing.

By changing yourself from the inside out, you will be able to attain and permanently maintain what I call your *get-real weight*. It is very important that I establish a clear definition in your mind of what this really means. Essentially, it means a weight that is healthy and realistic for your age and for your physical and genetic makeup, a weight at which you are happy and truly at peace with your size, and a weight that is stable because you have taken control of every factor in your life that keeps it there. Incidentally, that weight may not be at all what you now think you should weigh. For example, if you are a woman who is postmenopausal and you have had three children, and what you want is to be super-skinny like you were at age twenty-three, the reality is that you need to aim for something else. Your get-real weight is a state of health and well-being that is congruent and in harmony with how you are physically and genetically configured. It is the weight that is "right" for you—a stable, comfortable weight. It is the weight at which you look good, feel good, and lovingly accept yourself from the inside out.

THE SEVEN KEYS TO PERMANENT WEIGHT LOSS

What you are about to do to achieve your get-real weight will be unlike any diet or makeover program you have ever undertaken. I am going to give you seven critical pieces—I call them "keys"—to re-aligning and changing your life, internally and externally, in a way that will create, achieve, and maintain lasting weight loss.

Think about these keys in the following way: you are standing at the end of a long, up-sloped hallway with a series of seven locked doors, one after the other, all blocking your way to the other end. Each of the seven doors is a gateway, a through-way to specific, vital aspects of weight control. Up until now though, some of these doors have been locked to you. They've blocked your passage; they've been barriers to your success because you either have tried a dozen keys, all of them wrong, or you've failed to use every one of the right keys.

Only the right keys will do the trick. These are the keys I will give you in order to open each one of these doors—and to take the steps required to move down this hallway. When unlocked with the right keys, each of these seven doors will lead you closer to personal and permanent control over your weight. Obviously, your job is to unlock each door, step through it with a commitment to change, and keep moving forward until you've walked through all seven. Each step is an upward climb, and if you fail to unlock any door and step through it, you'll start rolling right back to where you started. Even if you go through two, or four, or six of the seven, you will be sucked right back to where you started, or worse. But if you make your way through all seven doors, at the end of your journey is everything you've ever wanted for yourself but have not been able to attain or maintain until now.

This book is about identifying those seven doors and giving yourself the seven keys to unlock them. Every person who reads this book should start from the same place. Some of the information may look familiar to you, but most of it won't. You may already have some of the keys and if so, great, we will focus on how to maximize what you have, building on and incorporating the foundation you have already laid. But many of you hold none of the keys. You haven't even opened the first door to permanent weight loss, and that is perfectly okay. This book is designed to meet you where you are. Even if you think you are familiar with a certain key, study it for reinforcement and encouragement, putting into action any additional steps that will build success and create value for you. Yes, you may have to spend more time on some keys than on others, but only by fully mastering all seven keys will you be able to do this right, this time, beginning now.

Yes, I realize that you'd love to go right to the part of this book in which I tell you what to eat or how to exercise. But it is this same sense of urgency and need for immediate gratification that has gotten you into trouble so many times before. Without going through the keys in sequence, you are likely to blow your chances of mastering them all. Be patient enough to do the work as outlined and you will prepare yourself for success. Resist the urge to jump ahead. You will get there soon enough, and when you do, you will get superior results.

Please keep this in mind too: the difference between those who can't keep their weight off and those who can is found in these seven keys. The 20 percent who fail to lose their weight long-term do not have or use all seven keys; the 80 percent who succeed, do. As one of my life laws states, "you either get it or you don't." The 80 percent get it. You are about to become one of those who gets it. We are going to land this plane!

Now for an overview of the seven keys.

KEY #1: RIGHT THINKING

In order for you to overcome your weight challenges, you have to first know exactly where you are starting. Where you are now with your weight struggles, everything you are, everything you do, begins with and is based on what I call your *personal truth*. By personal truth, I mean whatever it is about yourself and your weight problem that you have come to believe. This personal truth as it relates to your weight, and indeed to your entire life, is vitally important, because if you believe it, if it is real to you, then it is for you the precise reality you will live every day.

For instance, if you believe with utmost certainty that you will fail and never, ever, be able to manage your weight, then failure is what your personal truth dictates for you. What's more, your personal truth will show up as a heavy load of disgust, shame, guilt, hurt, self-hatred, and other self-critical voices that do nothing but drag you down. All of this gets incorporated into your deepest understanding of who you are and what you think you can accomplish, and it has the power to set you up for a specific outcome. And whatever your way of thinking, it provokes a physiological change. As a result of every thought you have, there is a corresponding physical reaction— reactions that may suppress your energy and prevent you from having what you truly want.

If your personal truth is riddled with counterproductive thoughts and beliefs, then my job, our job, is to get real about those parts of what you believe about yourself that aren't working for you, so that you can regain control over your weight. This is precisely what Key #1—right thinking—helps you do; it unlocks the door to *Self-Control*. Because your life is created from the inside out, you must first get right with yourself on the inside. With what you will learn and do here, you will put the past behind you, and confront your personal truth about your weight.

When you do this, you gain access to your real power, your real opportunity to impact your personal weight control. What this key enables you to do is discard all the toxic messages, replace them with realistic, positive thoughts, then act on this new, more constructive way of engaging the world.

Moving through this first door will be a challenging journey for you, one you have probably never undertaken because it means letting go of some long-standing and powerful forces in your life. But once you do this, once you step through this door, you will reclaim an incredible level of self-control. When you do the important work of this key, you will be able to fully and completely overwhelm your history and past negative momentum, and completely break the cycle of what it means to live as an overweight person.

KEY #2: HEALING FEELINGS

It is no big news flash that many people—you included—eat as a way to medicate themselves, usually in response to negative emotions such as anger, guilt, loneliness, stress, or boredom. You may also eat in response to positive emotions, such as happiness and joy, and in doing so you use food as a form of celebration. You have developed a strong emotional attachment to food, and this is one powerful reason why you turn to food when you crave love and emotional support. Emotional eating has figured hugely in your weight problem.

With the second key—healing feelings—you will unlock the door to *Emotional Control* and learn how to break the cycle of overeating in response to emotions and stress. You can't eliminate emotional triggers and stress—they're facts of life—but you can learn how to heal counterproductive responses to life's challenges and gain a new sense of control over your eating.

Glossing over this key, or denying that you have emotional issues with food, is a deal breaker. Your weight will never be lower or healthier unless and until you stop emotional overeating. This key helps you identify why you pursue emotional eating, and gives you a process, broken down in manageable steps, to unlock a newfound control over your eating behavior.

KEY #3: A NO-FAIL ENVIRONMENT

The third key unlocks the door to *External Control*, the ability to shape, design, and manage your environment so that it is virtually impossible for you to fail at weight control. With this key, you will concentrate on the personal landscape of your life that includes everything from your home to your office. You will focus on areas within this environment that must be "cleaned up" in order for you to lose weight.

This key is all about burning external bridges: minimizing opportunities that invite needless snacking, overeating, and bingeing; getting rid of the clothes of your plus-size life; and re-engineering your environment for success. With this key, you will do away with all reminders that could lessen your resolve and could, if you let them, fool you into thinking that it's much easier to go back to your former life. If you expect to succeed over the long haul, there is no regression or retreat to what you have always done before, or to what you have always been.

This key is amazing in that it will create immediate changes in how you act, think, live, and feel. With this key, you will make your life look different, feel different, and be different. When you begin to do different things, trust me, your actions will gain positive momentum. And through it all, you'll begin to feel better, more energized, and more focused mentally.

KEY #4: MASTERY OVER FOOD AND IMPULSE EATING

If you are stubbornly overeating, bingeing, or otherwise continuing in some repeated pattern of self-destructive habits and behaviors, discovering why you do this is not only worthwhile, it is essential to achieving permanent weight loss and control. With Key #4—mastery over food and impulse eating—you will unlock the door to *Habit Control*. Here, you will learn how to control and reshape your behavior, first by identifying why you persist in these bad habits, and second, by replacing them with actions designed to weaken their hold over you.

At some conscious, rational level, you know that it is counterproductive and extremely unhealthy to overeat, to binge, or to medicate yourself with food. But at some other level, these behaviors are rewarding you enough for you to keep doing them. Put another way, you are getting "payoffs" from your behavior. It is a law of life that "people do what works," and so your behaviors must work for you in some way. You are feeding some sort of need, or perhaps an aggregate of needs. As long as those needs are there, you will keep feeding them. While you continue to live like this, you reinforce habits and behaviors that become more difficult to weaken over time. Using this key, you will find and control the payoffs, unplug from those payoffs, and leave behind self-destructive behaviors.

We will also look at the specific ways you hurt your weight control efforts—the ways you interact with food that are in direct opposition to healthy behavior. You'll learn how to wipe bad, weight-gaining habits from your life and replace them with successful behaviors that will produce far more positive results. What's more, you'll find out how to manage your eating so that you are no longer controlled by impulses and urges. If—and only if—you can master this key, your personal control over your eating behavior will dramatically increase.

KEY #5: HIGH-RESPONSE COST, HIGH-YIELD NUTRITION

You are intelligent enough to know that if you take in more food than you burn off, you will gain unhealthy and unsightly amounts of weight. Yet you continue to choose the wrong foods in too-large amounts, putting taste and convenience ahead of nutrition and, as a result, no one has to shake the sheets to find you. The fifth key— high-response, high-yield nutrition—unlocks the door to *Food Control:* an approach to nutritional balance that is nothing short of revolutionary, and amazingly powerful in its simplicity.

There is no counting calories or grams, no measuring, no memorizing exhaustive food lists or exchanges. You will learn about food in a completely different context—in a way that no one, and no diet book, has ever discussed or previously put into widespread practice. This approach to nutrition is absolutely the most effective solution to managing food in your life. As you will find out, there are only two things you need to know about food—just two! With this key, you'll program your body to lose pounds and inches at a pace that is right for you. This is a key you can keep for a lifetime so that you can finally end your energy-draining battles with dieting and start living with a control over food you have not had in ages.

KEY #6: INTENTIONAL EXERCISE

Exercise is now counted as one of the top lifestyle factors to help you lose weight and keep it off for good. But the problem is, most people are so exercise-averse that they will never be in danger of drowning in their own sweat. If this description fits you, rest assured that I will not be asking you to spend endless hours in a gym, train to become an Olympic athlete, or grind yourself to the ground with boot camp-type calisthenics. Quite the contrary. With the sixth key, you will unlock the door to *Body Control*, the power to keep pounds at bay with a maximum-results workout strategy that you can start slowly and continue at your own pace.

One of the worst things I see with people trying to lose weight is that they become obsessive about exercise, so much so that this concern rises to a level of disordered, self-defeating behavior that can inflict a great deal of physical and psychological damage. Instead, you will be introduced to a balanced approach of simple strength-building and heart-conditioning exercises that provide a concentrated caloric burn. Yes, you will push yourself a little harder but you will feel amazed by what your body can do, and you'll feel so revitalized for doing it.

Using specific motivational tools, you will discover how to make exercise a focus of your energies—a permanent fixture in your life. This is a real chance for you to get control of your body, no matter how long it has been since you last exercised.

KEY #7: YOUR CIRCLE OF SUPPORT

Finally, using the seventh key, you will unlock the door to *Social Control*, with which you assemble a support circle of people who will encourage you and provide the accountability you need to achieve your goals. There is motivating energy in active, supportive ties to family and friends. If you want to truly lose weight, then you must try your best to surround yourself with a group of like-minded people who want you to do it, too. With these people in your life—your supporters—the more likely you are to succeed.

• • •

WARNING: because I know what you are probably thinking, I realize that some of these keys will not have "face validity" to you right now; they will not seem important to you on the surface. Some of the seven may seem "soft" or okay to gloss over. Do not make that mistake! Remember, the difference between those who keep it off, and those who don't, is that *they use all seven keys*. So if you are "really" sick to death of being overweight, if you have been fighting it for years, if you are tired of buying and wearing, pulling and tugging at a bunch of ugly "fat clothes," if you are fed up with failing, I mean really fed up, you can decide to change all of that right now—by using these keys to gain control of your weight, finally and permanently.

WHY THE SEVEN KEYS WORK WHEN OTHER PROGRAMS HAVE FAILED

There is no question that these keys provide an action-oriented plan to follow, one with verbs in the sentences. With each key, you will begin by focusing on defining and diagnosing where your behavior is now, with self-evaluations and assignments, because you will never be able to change what you do not acknowledge. Working interactively, you will get at what is mentally, emotionally, behaviorally, and socially not working in your life. Only when you figure out what your biggest obstacles are to weight control, can you match workable, livable solutions to them. All of this calls on you to play an active role. Once you have completed this important self-diagnosis, you will be given precise instructions—"steps through the door"—on what you need to do and how you need to do it, specific things you can do right away to begin generating results. And generate results now you will. This is not a plan in which two or three years from today you are at your goal weight and treading water to stay there. As soon as you start using the seven keys and following through on their action-filled steps, you will get right-now results; and you will be automatically setting up your world for long-term weight stability and maintenance.

You can free yourself forever from the bondage of your weight struggles, as long as you acquire the tools and stay accountable and action-oriented in making the important changes required. No one ever said that losing weight would be easy. Sticking with it can be challenging, but I have incredible news for you: the seven keys to permanent weight loss are designed to keep you going, even when you don't feel like doing so—and that's why they work when other programs have failed. They have as their foundation two essential motivational premises that afford you great power in losing weight and keeping it off for good. Here they are:

YOU DON'T NEED WILLPOWER

By now, you may have the impression that I will ask you to muster up "willpower" to master change. Wrong! Admit it: every time you ever started a new diet, you tried to white-knuckle it with willpower, didn't you? And the more you white-knuckled it, the more intensely you desired what you were resisting! You might be able to white-knuckle it for a while but you can't do it forever, because eventually you will cave in. This is a natural human impulse, and that's okay.

Let's get something straight: you have been lied to by the diet industry that you require willpower in order to successfully control your weight. You bought into that lie, and it has beaten you down, and crushed the very core of your being. You believed that you failed because you lacked sufficient willpower, and that somewhere inside you, you were weak and inadequate.

Okay, now comes something so liberating that you will wish that you had known it all along: you no longer need to rely on willpower. It simply doesn't work. Willpower is an outright myth, and your willingness to be deluded by this myth has sabotaged your weight-control efforts for far too long. Willpower is unreliable emotional fuel that drives you when you are excited, motivated, or energized. Willpower is what temporarily pumps you up when you want to lose weight in two weeks so you'll look good for a class reunion, or when you join a gym because you made a New Year's resolution to start exercising. At first, you feel like you're cooking on the front burner, as we say in Texas. But you know as well as I do, that no one stays fired up continuously, in fact, the burners are turned to the "off" position most of the time. Using willpower to achieve and sustain weight loss, or any lasting change for that matter, is destined for doom. The seven keys to permanent weight loss do not depend on willpower for success.

PROGRAM YOURSELF FOR SUCCESS

What they do depend on is programming—a far easier, much more effective, and practical way to sustain your commitment during those off times. Programming involves making small, deliberate modifications in the way you live your life, and it has everything to do with developing a lifestyle that creates healthier behavior.

I will go into a lot more detail later about programming, but let me give you some specific examples of what I am talking about. You program your life internally, from the inside out, so that you stop turning to food to mask feelings and medicate emotional distress. You program your life when you reduce your exposure to food by eliminating junk food from your kitchen. You program your life by cutting back on the time spent in the grocery store, or by minimizing the time it takes to prepare food. You program your life by arranging your schedule so that it easily accommodates exercise and activity. In short, you program your entire life for weight-control success—that means making it failure-proof—in order to manage your impulses, to set your life up for health and well-being, and to support you when the emotional energy of willpower isn't there to carry you through.

When you do these things, you set up a positive and powerful dominance in your life that absolutely and automatically both dictates immediate weight loss results and sustains them for the long term. With the right programming, you say good-bye to your old overweight self and begin to move toward a weight that is normal, stable, and healthy for you. Without programming, it is much harder to stay the course. Trust me, this method is a lot easier, and a whole lot more powerful, than counting on the fickle emotion of willpower.

With programming, along with the appropriate goals, actions, and self-management, you design your life so that it pulls for you when you're weak, when you're not pumped up, when you don't feel like behaving maturely, when you don't want to tell yourself "no." If you program yourself and your environment in such a way as to support your goals and actions, then you have programmed your world to help you lose weight, to sustain your commitment, and to live your life in a meaningful, purpose-driven way.

At this point, I don't expect you to know just yet what to do with each of the seven keys I have briefly described to you. In fact, I strongly suspect that you don't yet know the right questions to ask, let alone the answers. That's okay; we will do this together, so don't feel intimidated by the task ahead. You have a partner in me. A partner who is willing to guide you down the hallway, step by step, through each door. Along the way, I'm prepared to provide you with clear access to success-oriented steps and instructions on what you must do to have what you want. You have a partner who is willing to show you the way through this hallway and who will interact with you without wagging a finger, but with the willingness and courage to tell you the truth. I am going to be that guide and that partner for you. I will hand over to you the seven keys to permanent weight loss so that you can start losing weight and begin to live with renewed passion and power.

As soon as you begin to think, behave, and act differently, using these seven keys, your mind and body will reciprocate. Although it may be hard at first, you will discover that with each passing day, as you eat for health and nourishment, your addiction to refined sugar will grow so weak that it disappears. You will find that you are not fond of junk food, because it is "out of your system," both physically and psychologically. You will love the taste of real food again. You will not eat the whole box of Oreos. You will ask the waiter to doggy-bag the rest of the lasagna for lunch the next day. You will stop eating before you are full. No longer will you be obsessive about your weight. You will know what it is like not having to suck in your stomach or to camouflage your thighs. You will come to love your body, and live in it peacefully and comfortably. But more importantly, as you peel off your weight, you will take on a renewed, more alive way of being in the world, with the physical and emotional power to enjoy your life now and to its absolute fullest in your later years.

When you begin to take control of your weight in the coming weeks, I want you to know that it doesn't matter if you plan to lose 25, 50, 100, or 250 pounds. In fact, I do not want you to think too much about the number of pounds you want to lose. What I want you to focus on is requiring more of yourself, starting right now. Then and only then will those pounds come off. You can successfully accomplish this by consistently following the keys and the strategies I will give you here—and doing this one meal at a time, one day at a time, one step at a time. That is all I ask.

This is a good thing, really. Think about it: you can't predict the future, and you don't know what will happen tomorrow. You can deal only with the realities of the moment. It is when you look too far ahead, worrying about all the pounds you must lose, that you become overwhelmed, unfocused, and defeated. But if you concentrate on the here and now, the present moment, believe me, your weight will come off.

I also want to impress upon you that valuable and limited time is going to slip away whether or not you decide to take up these keys. My father used to tell me, "When you kill time, remember you can't resurrect it." So I can assure you, at this precise time next year, your weight will be higher or lower than it is right now. It will not be the same; the choice to reduce it or let it pile higher and higher is entirely and unquestionably yours.

So please: don't say you will start on this tomorrow, or on Monday, or even later today. Decide this very moment whether you will use the seven keys to permanent weight loss. It could be the single most significant decision you make to maximize the quality of your health and change the direction of your life.

To point you in that direction, we are first going to look at how to set reasonable and realistic goals for change, goals that will help you use the seven keys to their fullest advantage, so that you not only lose your unwanted weight but learn to live a healthier, fuller life from this point forward.

2

Get-Real Expectations and Goals

Even I don't wake up looking like Cindy Crawford.
—CINDY CRAWFORD

There she sat in my counseling office, her face streaming with tiny rivulets of tears, her voice quivering between sobs. She placed three photographs of herself across my desk like a hand of solitaire, all from her high school days, showing a body so thin that she could walk through a harp and not strike a note. "If only I could lose weight and be thin again, I'd be so happy. I want to lose this weight so badly. I want to look like these pictures again, but I can't."

And so here was Catherine, a woman who was clearly 60 to 70 pounds overweight, trying desperately to diet down to her high school weight, only to watch the scales climb higher and higher because she was never successful at reaching her goal, or even coming close. She yearned to understand why her body would not cooperate; why, despite jumping through fad-diet hoops, her figure would not return to that of her teenage years. Why, why, why? At the same time, she believed that if she could only reach this idealized goal weight, then all her troubles would vanish with her excess pounds.

In counseling sessions and in seminars across the country, I have heard this same sad story thousands of times from thousands of people. They want desperately to get skinny, so skinny, in fact, that they'd have to stand up twice to cast a shadow. They want to be as scarce-hipped as the media models whose images have overstimulated their senses from every direction. They will go to extreme measures, from starving to purging, in their pursuit of thinness. With barely a morsel passing between their lips, they relentlessly try to strip their bodies of fat, and if they don't drop five pounds in a week on one diet, they move on to another, trying to mold themselves into the illusion of society's image of the perfect body. (I'm talking to men here, too. You aren't totally immune either. It's no longer enough for you to make it in the world; now you think you have to look the part too—muscled and youthful, with movie-hero good looks.)

And they really and truly think that losing weight will solve all of life's problem. Reality check: you can never, ever, use weight loss to solve problems that are not related to your weight. At your goal weight or not, you still have to live with yourself and deal with your problems. You will still have the same husband, the same job, the same kids, and the same life. Losing weight is not a cure for life.

But know this: if you faithfully use the seven keys to weight loss, you will have a greater sense of mastery over your entire life. You will be different, with more coping energy, a clearer focus, and a reordered lifestyle. You will be in a much better position to handle life's ups and downs, because you will have rendered null and void all the ways you destructively think, feel, and act. You will be living the life you desire and deserve.

In order to make that happen, what you must begin to do is stop dealing with fairy-tale fantasies about your weight and your life, and instead help yourself get in touch with certain factual realities about yourself so that you can attain permanent weight loss. As we go through this chapter together, you must be willing to challenge the reality that you may want and pursue things in regard to your weight that simply aren't right for you. This means that you will have to get real about where you are right now and what you can reasonably achieve. Being able to go after your goals with a *realistic expectation* that you will achieve them is of great relevance to your ability to lose weight and keep it off. Why? If you have unrealistic expectations, you can and will fail.

Once you wake up to this truth, you'll stop saying to yourself, I have to look a certain way, I have to be perfect, I have to do this or that. Rather, you'll say, I will do what works for me, I will adjust my life to what is best for my health and my well-being, and I will make the right changes in order to be in harmony with reality.

Let me interject something important here, before we move on:

if there is one thing I know after thirty years of working with people who have weight problems, it's that you might feel such a sense of urgency to get started on the seven keys that you're willing to run through a brick wall. But you would cheat yourself terribly if you try to skip this chapter and plow ahead. Seeking after "I want it now" immediate gratification, when you are excited and your emotional energy is high, has been the cause of more failed attempts at weight loss than I could ever begin to describe. You need to work on building the right mind-set in order to get on and stay on the right track. You are going to tap into some insights here that will help you make powerful changes in your ability to manage your weight. So all I ask is that you spend the twenty minutes it takes to read this chapter. Focus on what you need to do here, and it will guide you toward what you want.

So together, let's begin to bring into focus the true, the authentic "you" and everything you are capable of achieving.

REALISTIC EXPECTATIONS

Maybe you are not suffering from the obsessive diet and thought patterns that I described at the beginning of this chapter, at least not yet. But I'm willing to bet that you don't like your body much, that you have a poor "body image," and this is setting you up for trouble down the road.

Before I go any further, let me explain this concept of body image to you, which applies to both men and women. It's best that you don't think of body image as what you see when you look in the mirror; it's a reaction you have within you in response to what you see. Body image encompasses the things you tell yourself about how you look, good or bad, fat or thin, good-looking or ugly, and whether you are satisfied or dissatisfied with what you see when you see yourself in the mirror.

How you feel about your body can have a dramatic effect on your *self-concept*—a more inclusive term that describes the bundle of beliefs, facts, judgments, and perceptions you have about yourself, every moment of the day. What you believe about your body shapes your self-concept and how it gets expressed, to some extent. If you don't like your body, this self-rejection is likely to weaken your self-concept and make you feel that you can never be worthwhile.

On the other hand, accepting and loving your body makes you feel better about yourself and what you can accomplish. It makes you feel more confident that you can lose weight and better control the course of your health. So your body image is a big, big deal.

MAXIMIZE THE BEST YOU

If you have a poor body image, there is a high likelihood that you are passively allowing the media, and perhaps other people in your world, to shape your body image, and this can begin to poison your self-concept. Maybe you've bought into the worn-out cliché, "You can never be too rich or too thin." When that happens, the pursuit of an unattainable ideal ultimately can become so embedded in the fiber of your being that it consumes you.

If you are judging your body against the media images of beautiful people who are touched up, airbrushed up, pushed up, and whatever elsed-up, you are not living in the real world. In real life you do not go around dressed in couture clothes, your skin is not flawless, and not every hair is in place. Unlike the pictures in the magazines, you do have cellulite on your thighs, you do have a spare tire around your waist, your roots do show, and you do have freckles and age spots. And sure, a lot of times you do look pretty great, you do turn heads, but get real, there are those days when you look like ten miles of bad road. You are living in the real world here.

If you are truly out of shape and you don't like it, then having a negative body image may mean that you are taking a realistic view of yourself—a good thing, actually. It's only a problem if you don't work to improve it. So the fact that you don't like what you see in the mirror is a powerful catalyst for becoming fitter, healthier, and better looking. You can't heal what you don't acknowledge. Admitting to yourself what is wrong about your body is a positive. In the past, you may have treated this kind of admission as a negative. But that attitude is for losers. It's choosing denial, instead of reality, and it will keep you from taking corrective action. On the other hand, when you acknowledge the truth about yourself, shortcomings and all, but without beating up on yourself unnecessarily, this prompts you to take important and timely steps toward change. It sends you on your way to creating a new, healthier experience.

What I want you to guard against, though, is setting standards for yourself that are unattainable. If you are striving for a perfection that doesn't exist, because there is no perfection, you have set up such an unreal expectation that you are living in a dream world. You are pursuing a fantasy that is incongruent with who you are, and this pursuit can chip away at your body image.

God brought us all into this world in a pleasing array of diverse shapes and sizes, and we are genetically programmed to be a certain way: tall, short, muscular, stout, or thin as a fiddle string. Your unique physical traits and characteristics, your height, your musculature, and your bone structure are what define your physical being and appearance, and differentiate you from every other human being in the world. There has never been another you in the history of the world, and there never will be. You are uniquely designed and gifted, with a core purpose for being in this world. That was God's plan, and for you to reject that and say, "I'm not good enough for me" is not okay.

At this very moment, you may be saying to yourself that you have any number of admirable qualities. You are a loyal friend, a caring person, someone who is smart, dependable, fun to be around. That's wonderful, and I'm happy for you, but let me ask you this: are you being any of those things to yourself? I always say that the most important relationship you will ever have is with yourself. You've got to be your own best friend first, accepting and loving yourself from the inside out, before you can be truly happy and before you can live with purpose and passion. Once you start appreciating your body, trust me, you will begin to take much better care of yourself, and you will find that weight loss is so much easier because you are treating yourself with respect.

One of the most powerful ways to attain a more positive body image is to have realistic expectations about what you can achieve and then to set realistic goals to achieve them. That's why you must factor your genetics and God-given physical attributes into your personal goal setting. I had an aunt who was tall enough to hunt geese with a garden rake—6 feet, 5 inches, actually, with a very large bone structure. Her hands were as big as hams. She weighed 220 pounds—huge by most standards—but here's the clincher: she had barely an ounce of fat on her body, probably no more than 10 percent, she was the right weight for her structure and genetics.

That is why it is important for you to take stock of who you are and how you are physically and genetically configured. If you are a woman and what you want is to look like Cindy Crawford, or if you are a man and what you want is to look like Pierce Brosnan, but you're short and on the stocky side, the chances are that you need to want something else.

WHAT IS YOUR GET-REAL WEIGHT?

If you have realistic expectations about what you should rightfully achieve for good health, then you are very likely going to succeed in your efforts and make peace with your body because you will be living in concert with realistic goals. That's why I have to bring up the subject of what is the healthiest, most realistic weight for you—your get-real weight—because I know this is on your mind. There are two ways of looking at your get-real weight, medically and psychologically, and I am going to address both because they are of equal and related importance.

Medically, there is a healthy weight for you—one that is realistic for your physical and genetic makeup—and we have to talk about this because your health is at stake. You are probably wondering, "What, then, should I realistically weigh?"

There are numerous methods you can use to determine a realistic goal weight, none without inherent flaws. For example, many of the height-weight tables are based on oversimplified, obsolete formulas created more than twenty years ago. The ideal weights they propose are too heavy for short people, and impossibly low for very tall men and women. Take me, for example. I'm 6 feet, 4 inches, and large-boned. Those tables suggest that I should weigh about 181. At that weight, you could use me for a clothesline.

The same holds true for another measurement called the "Body Mass Index" (BMI), which employs your weight and height to judge the amount of fat you have on your body. Even so, BMI is not an accurate method for assessing your weight. For example, it is unreliable for women who are pregnant or breast-feeding, chronically ill patients, exercisers, competitive athletes, and bodybuilders. In fact, if you measured Arnold Schwarzenegger using this method, he would be labeled "obese" because BMI doesn't distinguish between fat and muscle (muscle weighs more than fat), and you certainly don't want to tell Arnold that he's fat!

Sizes of men and women have been gradually increasing over time. People are just naturally heavier now than they were twenty years ago, so none of these methods of calculating a realistic goal is really usable, nor are they applicable. Working with overweight patients, I used two systems: *Body Shape Standards* and *Body Weight Standards*, to help them set their get-real weight goals.

Body Shape Standards helped my patients monitor their shape by periodically determining their "waist-to-hip ratio." This is important because weight distribution—where you carry weight on your body—can affect your health, for better or for worse. The distribution of excess body fat is commonly categorized as "apple type" or "pear type." Apple body types store excess fat in their stomach region, and are at greater risk for heart disease, diabetes, and certain cancers. Pear body types store excess fat around their hips and thighs and are at risk for joint problems and obesity, with its slew of health risks.

Calculating your waist-to-hip ratio is easy:

- Using a tape measure, measure your waist at your belly button.

- Measure your hips at their widest point. (Stand with your feet apart, in a relaxed position.)

- Divide your waist measurement by your hip measurement to arrive at your waist-to-hip ratio.

Ideally, this number should be 0.80 or less if you are a woman; or 0.95 or less if you are a man. As you lose weight, you'll reduce and redistribute your body fat, leading to a lower waist-to-hip ratio.

The other tool, Body Weight Standards, is a system I formulated for my patients. It is a modified and more realistic version of height-weight tables. Though not perfect, these body weight standards are more reflective of what can be achieved, and certainly a better measure of where most people should be, weight-wise.

Use the Body Weight Standards, listed in the table below, to help identify some targets so that you can move forward from where you are now. The lower end of the ranges are for small-boned people; the upper end, for larger-boned individuals. Be honest here: don't subjectively say you are small-boned, when in fact you are just the opposite.

TABLE 1.
DR. PHIL'S BODY WEIGHT STANDARDS*

HEIGHT	WOMEN	MEN
4' 10"	90–100–110	114–127–140
4' 11"	95–105–116	119–132–145
5'	99–110–121	123–137–151
5' 1"	103–115–127	128–142–156
5' 2"	108–120–132	132–147–162
5' 3"	112–125–138	137–152–167
5' 4"	117–130–143	141–157–173
5' 5"	122–135–148	146–162–178
5' 6"	126–140–154	150–167–184
5' 7"	130–145–160	155–172–189
5' 8"	135–150–165	159–177–195
5' 9"	139–155–171	164–182–200
5' 10"	144–160–176	168–187–206
5' 11"	148–165–182	173–192–211
6'	153–170–187	177–197–217
6' 1"	157–175–193	182–202–222
6' 2"	162–180–198	186–207–228
6' 3"	166–185–204	191–212–233
6' 4"	171–190–209	195–217–239

* *Weight in pounds.*

Psychologically, though, your get-real weight has little to do with numbers on a scale or other device. It means:

- You like your body and live in it with pride.

- You are happy and truly at peace with your size.

- You accept your God-given uniqueness.

- You treat your body with respect, care, and love.

- You like what you see in the mirror every day.

- You focus your attention on living well, rather than looking good.

So, lovingly accept yourself, your natural body frame, your height, your bone structure, your entire genetic makeup—and set your sights on goals that match these factual realities, goals that you can realistically achieve. There is an optimal you, but it can only come from getting real about yourself and setting realistic expectations for success, so that you can become a "supermodel" or "superstar" in your own life, on your own terms, and according to your own standards of fitness.

GET-WITH-IT GOAL SETTING

If you've been frustrated because you never seem to reach your weight loss goal, or stay at your goal weight, one reason may be that you have not yet learned how to set goals with any degree of specificity, or you've aimed for unrealistic, pie-in-the-sky stuff that you couldn't reach no matter how hard you tried. Failure to set specific, realistic goals makes your journey toward your destination like that of an unguided missile, an approach that simply will not work and will miss the mark every time.

For you to achieve what you want, when you want it, you must have realistic weight goals in focus, with specifically defined actions for reaching them. Don't just wake up every morning and react to what happens. Please don't do that. Be proactive by setting goals and making plans for their attainment. Goal setting is not something you do when you feel like it, because if you do, you will lose your momentum and your sense of purpose with regard to your weight.

What I'm about to tell you about goal setting may be information you've never heard before, so pay super-close attention. With weight management, goals are generally expressed in terms of the pounds you want to lose or the weight you want to reach—and those are worthwhile, specific goals. These goals are critical to the goal-setting process, and you need to set them. They have motivating merit, because they keep your momentum moving in a positive direction.

What happens once you've reached that goal, once you've dropped the 20, 30, 50, or 100 pounds you wanted to lose? Now what? Have you changed anything else in your life that will help you maintain your weight loss? Your sense of motivation and momentum could come to a grinding halt, if all you aimed for was the loss of X number of pounds. The weight is gone, but the need for new behaviors to sustain that weight loss still remains. Changing behaviors and programming your world for success provide the additional impetus that will help you keep those pounds off. So there is more to weight loss goals than just the number of pounds you want to weigh.

When people go after goals, they typically confuse the means with the end. They focus on an object or an end event, such as the weight they want to reach, without ever following through to the next important step, which is identifying how being at that weight would make them feel. Let's use the example of pounds again. You might define your goal in these terms: "I want to weigh 125 pounds." I would suggest to you that weighing 125 pounds is a means to an end, rather than the end in itself. You need to go further. You must be willing to ask yourself, "*Why* do I want to weigh 125 pounds?"

For one thing, are you doing it because your spouse, your parents, or somebody else in your life wants you to? Are you intent on pleasing them? Because if you are, you need to rethink this whole deal. When the priorities are someone else's, and not your own, you're spending all your precious time and energy working for external approval, trying to please other people by meeting their expectations while ignoring your own. You'll be miserable because you are denying what is genuinely important to you. You can't make other people happy—life doesn't work that way—but you can make yourself happy. That said, the question remains: "Why do you want to weigh 125 pounds?"

The real answer is very likely that you want to achieve that weight because of *how you think you will feel when you get there.* In this example, weighing 125 pounds represents for you the idea that you will look good and feel better at a smaller size, something you probably desire very strongly. Your ultimate goal, then, is not only weighing 125 pounds, but also having the specific feelings attached to that weight.

This is an important distinction. If you can recognize that it's not just the specific weight you want to attain, but also the *feelings* that you associate with it, then your goal expands from the weight to the connected emotions. If you can come to realize that what you really want is to feel better about yourself, then your goal also becomes the feeling.

You can look at this another way: if what you really want is to feel better about yourself, it would be unfair to restrict yourself to one method—like a diet—to get there. Maybe there are many different ways for you to arrive at the same destination—exercising, cutting out junk foods, doing relaxation exercises when you feel the urge to binge—and any one of these behaviors would help you lose weight and feel better about yourself. Your chances of getting what you want, when you have so many avenues of pursuit, are clearly greater than when you've limited those methods to just one or two. Not coincidentally, the seven keys to permanent weight loss all give you multiple paths to achieve a weight that is right for you.

You need to know so much about what you want, that when you are heading toward it, you know it, feel it, sense it. When you know a goal intimately, you'll feel it when you get close. As with a diamond, a goal is multifaceted, with many different points and sides. So when I say that you must have intimate knowledge of what you want, I mean that you must be able to describe your goals in a variety of terms and from different points of view. When you know what you want—how it looks, how it feels, and what experiences it contains—then you can begin to guide your life like a ship toward the harbor light because you now have goals that are exactly, precisely, and realistically defined.

SET YOUR GOALS

Because I have counseled so many overweight patients, I can tell you with absolute certainty why some people stay fit and others do not. If someone is successful in keeping weight off for five, ten, twenty, or more years, they have carefully planned, thoughtful goals that they hold to and live by. Without question, it is this focused, goal-oriented approach to life that distinguishes winners from losers. It is a common denominator present among all winners, from every walk of life and in every endeavor of life including weight management. Having specific, carefully mapped out, vividly envisioned goals is an absolute requirement for success. Without such goals, you will fail.

But the good news is that when you employ the goal-setting strategy I will give you here, you will get what you want because you will know exactly, precisely, what it is that you want. You will be able to see it, feel it, and experience it in your mind, in your heart, and in your spirit. You will be able to envision it so clearly that you can project yourself forward to that time of victory, of living and being in a new body, with renewed energy, renewed vigor, and a renewed way of being in the world. You will be able to describe it as though you were living it today. You will know what "fit and healthy" looks like and feels like, and how it will change your life.

Now, if you're ready to start generating great results that will distinguish you from the crowd and make you a winner, it is time to map out your goals in terms of five multidimensional criteria. What follows are some simple yet critical guidelines for setting, following, and attaining your goals. You'll learn how to define and describe your goals in meaningful and motivating ways. This section is interactive too; I will provide the guidelines, and you will fill in the blanks that correspond to each guideline. It is super-important to write this information down too, so that you can visually anchor your goal-setting strategy. Vividly envisioned goals, written down, allow you to stay on course and get closer to the finish line.

Express your goals in terms of specific behaviors and feelings.

One of the greatest difficulties with goals is that they are often poorly defined, murky, and without sufficient detail. For example, if you say, "I'm going to lose weight," then your goal isn't very helpful because it's too fuzzy. This kind of goal setting practically ensures failure; it doesn't tell how you will lose weight.

The most effective and motivating goals are those that describe *behavioral change*—in other words, what will be done. Thus, a better goal statement might be: "I intend to lose weight by getting to the gym four times a week and by following the food plan in this book." By describing your goals in terms of specific behaviors—exercising and eating right—you can go after them more directly and successfully than you could an ambiguous, blue-sky statement like "I want to lose weight." Only when your goals are specific, and focus on changing behaviors, will your attempts at losing weight and keeping it off be successful.

As I have mentioned, the other important facet of goal setting asks, "How will you feel when you achieve your goal?" That too must be answered with specificity. For example, if you want to feel the peace that derives from losing weight, be specific about what you mean by "peace." Does it mean an absence of chaotic overeating, freedom from on-again, off-again dieting, an active lifestyle that promotes physical harmony? You can use the space below to define and describe your goal in this manner.

With specificity, write what it is you hope to achieve (the number of pounds you want to lose or the desire to maintain your weight loss within a certain range once you have lost it):

_____

_____

_____

_____

Describe what you will do (the behaviors or actions you must commence, change, or stop in order to lose weight):

_____

_____

_____

_____

When you lose weight, you want to feel (proud of your new shape, lighter, more energetic, free from obsessions over food or dieting, at peace with your body, and so forth):

_____

_____

_____

_____

_____

Footnote: this aspect of targeting behaviors for change as a part of your goal-setting strategy is all-important for achieving permanent weight loss. Understand that it is not possible for you to be overweight unless you have generated and adopted a lifestyle to sustain it. You have set up that lifestyle, based upon numerous self-destructive behaviors such as overeating, bingeing, not exercising, and self-defeating internal dialogue, that have contributed to and sustained your weight problem. You have set up your world to keep yourself overweight, even though you consciously confess that you want to be fit, energetic, and of normal weight. You make sure your life revolves around food. If you are chronically overweight, I know that your manner of living can be characterized as inert, harried, and chaotic. You do not exercise; you are not a member of a gym or if you are, you haven't actually graced the doors of one in ages, and quite predictably, your main leisure time activity is watching television. Even your internal and emotional reactions are keeping your weight-sustaining lifestyle alive. Yes, you have set up your world and chosen your lifestyle in a way that supports staying overweight. You have chosen to live in a way in which no other result could occur.

But when you honestly acknowledge these behaviors, as you did above, you have targeted them for change. Remember, you cannot change what you do not acknowledge. And when you change these behaviors using the seven keys, when you abandon these negative parts of your lifestyle, your weight will take care of itself. With each of the seven keys, you will be able to deconstruct your world, internally and externally, and put it back together with a new lifestyle that gives you long-lasting change and permanent weight loss and control.

Express your goal(s) in terms that can be measured and are realistic.

Your weight loss goals must be expressed in terms of outcomes that are measurable—and realistic. In order for something to rise to the level of a measurable, realistic goal, you've first got to be able to quantify it by attaching a realistic number to it.

Returning to the example of "I want to lose weight," you would define that goal with the same kind of specificity stated above (the behaviors and feelings associated with reaching that goal), but also in terms that are measurable. That is, you'd express your goal in such a way that it has a clear outcome. For example, you might say, "I intend to lose 50 pounds to reach my goal weight of 125 pounds."

This dimension of measurability is pivotally important because it helps you monitor your progress toward your goals. You need to know how much of the goal you've attained, whether you're approaching it, how far you still have to go, and whether you've attained your goal or not. In the above example, you can easily measure your progress toward that goal by weighing yourself on a scale each week.

This goal-setting technique is valuable when applied to behaviors such as exercising. Let's say you want to revamp and organize your lifestyle in such a way that there is always time for exercise. In order to do this, you might express an exercise goal like this: "I will briskly walk three miles a day, four times a week, every week, in the morning before work." Walking three miles a day, four times a week, every week, is a goal that can be measured. Further, you have attached a specific time slot to your exercise session—*in the morning before work*—and this makes your goal all the more specific and keeps you efficiently on track. Or you might do this: set a goal to walk 10,000 steps a day, a number now recommended by physicians for controlling weight and building fitness. Purchase a pedometer, a device you can attach to your belt or pocket that, when activated, measures the exact number of steps you take over the course of a day.

When you can measure an outcome, your chances of success go

way, way up. You see, in concrete detail, how close you are to achieving your goal. There is reinforcement and motivating power that comes with seeing yourself succeed like this.

Red alert: when you describe your goals as measurable, quantifiable outcomes, let me remind you that they must be realistic. If you want to lose weight and keep it off, you must hold yourself to realistic expectations, not setting weight goals that are impossible to achieve. Do not say you will get down to the size 4 of your youth, when you know that is unrealistic. Know what you can realistically achieve and maintain, and set your goals from that truth.

Review what you have already written regarding your goals. In the space below, express your goals in terms of measurable outcomes, such as how many pounds you want to lose and what weight you'd like to achieve. Again, make sure this weight is realistic for your height and bone structure; refer back to the Body Weight Standards table (page 28) for guidance.

_____

_____

_____

Assign a timeline to your goal.

To achieve what you envision, your goals require a particular schedule or calendar for their achievement. Unless you attach a schedule to your goals, they become nothing more than dreams or fantasies floating around in your head. Once you say when you want to achieve a carefully defined goal in a carefully defined time frame, that goal takes on greater significance, with stronger forward momentum. If you've decided your initial goal is to lose 50 pounds in twenty-five weeks, your date would be twenty-five weeks from the day you start. Working backward from that date, you can see where you need to be at the midpoint of twelve weeks. Likewise, you can see where you have to be at the five-week mark and two-week mark.

Recognize that as you go through this countdown toward your goal, you will experience inevitable plateaus. These are points along the way at which your weight loss will slow down or appear to stop or taper off as your metabolism shifts to accommodate your new healthier size. You may feel like the "slow-mo" button has been hit, causing your weight loss to go into a foot-dragging mode. Don't be alarmed or get so frustrated that you throw in the towel; this is only your body making physiological adjustments. It does not mean you have stopped losing weight. As long you stay focused and action-oriented, you will bulldoze right over these plateaus.

As you map out a time line, thinking in terms of a calendar allows you to assess the realism of your plan, and to determine the intensity of what you must do to reach your goal. So once you have determined precisely what you want, you must decide on a time line for having it. In the space below, create a time line for achieving your goal. Transfer this information to your calendar or daily planner.

_____

_____

_____

_____

_____

_____

_____

Break down your goal into manageable steps.

Most people express their weight loss goals with statements such as, "I'm going to fit into size 6 jeans, down from a size 18" or "I'm going to lose 50 pounds in the New Year." Those are what I call "dream world statements" because, if you think about it, they describe a fantasy of what you want to look like. Don't get me wrong; fantasizing about what you want to look like is an important step toward genuine change for the better. But if you want to make change happen, you have to turn that dream into reality by defining a realistic goal, carefully broken down into workable, measurable steps attached to a time line, as we discussed above. So instead of saying you are going to fit into size 6 jeans by summer, it is more reasonable and effective to express your goal in these terms: "I will take certain steps to lose two pounds a week for the next twenty-five weeks. At the end of that time, I will be able to fit into size 6 jeans."

Weight loss doesn't just happen; it happens one step at a time.

Considered in its entirety, the thought of losing 50 pounds and dropping several sizes can be so overwhelming that it is paralyzing. But it begins to look doable when broken down into manageable steps. The steps you determine may be as simple as:

I will use the keys in this book and follow the action steps presented.

I will walk four times a week for one hour each time.

I will eliminate junk food from my diet.

I will productively and positively manage the stress in my life in order to stop overeating in response to stressful events.

Know what your steps will be. As you learn about each key to permanent weight loss, come back to here and add other steps required to reach your goals. In the space below, record the steps involved in reaching your goal:

I will take certain steps to reach my goal weight. These steps are as follows:

Create accountability.

Have a trusted, loyal checkpoint person in your life to whom you require yourself to report on your progress. This person may be a family member, your spouse, or your best friend. At least once a week, check in with this person and report on your compliance toward reaching your goals. In the space below, list some individuals who might be helpful in this role.

_____

_____

_____

_____

Before leaving this all-important subject of goal setting, let me emphasize that life moves by momentum. If you are overeating, not exercising, slumping on your couch every night with a beer in one hand and chips in the other, what you are doing is a product of negative momentum, building in speed and intensity toward failure unless that momentum is reversed.

The goals you set for yourself, and the way you describe and define them, are critical to reversing that negative momentum so that you succeed for the long haul. You must be driven in just such a way to shed pounds, keep them shed, and live your life in a healthy, positive way. That is your priority. You must hold yourself to higher standards now. You cannot be wishy-washy about your decision to get your weight under control, and you can't run hot and cold from one day to the next. You can't allow yourself to test the waters just to see how it goes. Tentativeness and playing it safe never get you anywhere. Your goals should allow for no second-guessing.

A tried and true formula fits here: BE—DO—HAVE. BE committed, DO what it takes, and you will HAVE what you want. Don't decide to work toward your goals just for some preset period of time. You have to commit to pursuing your goals, using the seven keys, "until." You work on this until you have what you want.

From here forward, your life will be focused upon, energized by, and defined in relation to the goals you have set. You will know what you want, and you will evaluate each and every option in your life against the priority of your goals. Make the resolve to be committed, know that you are special and that your goals are worth having, and when you achieve them, step up and claim your right to have them.

3

Are You Ready?

*If you care enough for a result, you will most
certainly attain it.*
—WILLIAM JAMES

It is now estimated that roughly 65 percent of our population is
overweight—an epidemic! Now considered the leading cause of pre-
ventable death in America (smoking is number two), obesity is acknowledged as one of the medical conditions most resistant to
permanent treatment—even harder to treat than cancer, by many accounts. If you're like most people who go on diets, you will regain
your lost weight after one year, and very few of you will ever achieve
lasting weight loss.

If you're overweight or obese, you're putting your health on the
line. You are at the highest risk of heart disease, stroke, some cancers,
type II diabetes, gallbladder problems, arthritis, and early death. That
means a whole lot of you are barreling toward a medical disaster and
cheating yourself out of longevity. Surely, you do not want to be part
of this herd of statistics, do you?

I certainly hope not, but let's begin to find out right here. Let's
find out if you are ready to embrace a new kind of thinking, a new
way of looking at yourself, a new way of living—one that will result
in lasting weight loss. Will you refuse to be a part of the epidemic in
America that is turning us into a nation of fatties? Will you? Are you
ready to unlock the doors to permanent weight loss? Are you?

There is an old joke in psychology: how many psychologists does
it take to change a light bulb? Answer: only one, but the light bulb
has to want to change. People change only when they are ready, and
you need to find out the exact state of your readiness for change.
That is why I want you take the following test called *Your Readiness
Profile* before you begin to use the seven keys. Answer all the ques-

tions honestly, take as much time as you need, and be sure to pay close attention to the interpretation of your score.

YOUR READINESS PROFILE

Answer the following questions by marking *Yes*, *Undecided*, or *No*.

1. I am ready to eat differently even if it hurts my family's or my friends' feelings, or causes conflict.

   Yes ( )   Undecided ( )   No ( )

2. I am ready to throw away clothes that are too big and no longer fit me.

   Yes ( )   Undecided ( )   No ( )

3. I am ready to temporarily give up any friends who do not totally support me and who may wish to sabotage my weight-management efforts.

   Yes ( )   Undecided ( )   No ( )

4. I am at the end of my rope, and I know that I have nowhere to go but up at this point; I am willing to focus totally using the seven keys.

   Yes ( )   Undecided ( )   No ( )

5. I admit that I have been unsuccessful in trying to manage my weight in the past, either by following a diet or some other program, but that I am willing to follow the steps and strategies outlined in this book.

   Yes ( )   Undecided ( )   No ( )

6. I am willing to read this book and honestly use the keys in order to change myself, my lifestyle, and my behavior.

   Yes ( )   Undecided ( )   No ( )

7. I am willing to look at my behavior honestly and answer to myself and other significant people in my life about my problems.

   Yes ( )   Undecided ( )   No ( )

8. I am willing to confront myself and others honestly about how I sabotage myself or allow myself to get sabotaged.

Yes ( )   Undecided ( )   No ( )

9. I am willing to change my job, if necessary, to become healthier and manage my weight better.

Yes ( )   Undecided ( )   No ( )

10. I am willing to throw away all the problem food in my house and eat according to the food and behavioral steps and strategies outlined in this book.

Yes ( )   Undecided ( )   No ( )

11. I am willing to exercise at least three to four hours a week at a moderate level of effort.

Yes ( )   Undecided ( )   No ( )

12. I am willing to make my health and the control of my weight a top priority in my daily life.

Yes ( )   Undecided ( )   No ( )

13. I am willing to dedicate at least fifteen to twenty minutes a day in focused concentration to follow the weight-management steps in this book.

Yes ( )   Undecided ( )   No ( )

14. I am willing to give myself self-affirmations the majority of the time to overturn negative thinking.

Yes ( )   Undecided ( )   No ( ) .

15. I am willing to talk straight about what I am doing, and not fool myself into thinking that anyone else can do this for me but me.

Yes ( )   Undecided ( )   No ( )

16. I am willing to stop lying to myself, and to others, about things that blind me from being who I am.

Yes ( )   Undecided ( )   No ( )

17. I am willing to transform these steps into action by using the seven keys and not dropping out because "it is too hard" or because "I am not strong enough."

Yes ( )   Undecided ( )   No ( )

18. I am willing to admit that I have some problems, but that I will not let these problems damage my commitment to the steps and strategies in this book.

Yes ( )   Undecided ( )   No ( )

19. I admit that I must take responsibility for my life, and I am committed to making permanent changes.

Yes ( )   Undecided ( )   No ( )

20. I am willing to say out loud to myself that I will change my lifestyle for better health.

Yes ( )   Undecided ( )   No ( )

SCORING

Count only the "yeses" and add them together for a score of 0 to 20.

INTERPRETING YOUR SCORE:

0 to 3: Comfort Zone

If your score is this low, then we have to talk because you've taken a padded seat in a dangerous place called the comfort zone. That means you are not yet ready to change—in fact you are far from it, and this book will do you no good at this point. You are avoiding reaching for any level of change that is not already comfortable. At some level, it is quite possible that you are in denial, resistant even to confronting your problem. If you are, you respond with statements such as:

My weight doesn't really bother me.

I've always been on the heavy side.

My husband likes me this way.

I think fat is beautiful.

If you pretend that the way you are is okay and you rationalize why you don't want to change and have more, there is no risk of failure and the discouragement that goes along with it. You accept what you've got and play it safe. In reality though, you have settled for what you don't really want, for a very rational—if unproductive—reason. By taking a seat in the comfort zone, you remove yourself from the fear of reaching and possibly failing.

While comfortable, that sort of life can be more than inert. Staying in your comfort zone can be hazardous to your health and your genuine well-being. If your lifestyle is riddled with bad behavior, wrong thinking, and poor choices—and you don't do something about it—you are staring at our country's top killers: heart disease, cancer, diabetes, and other serious diseases. You have the primary responsibility for initiating change in your life. If your weight problem is to change, it will be because you changed the way you think, feel, and do. Get out of your seat in the comfort zone and resolve to begin each and every day of your life with the question: What can I do to get healthy control of my weight and my life? Ask it, answer it, then do it, every day.

4 to 10: Fence-Sitting

If this was your score, you are straddling the fence, which means you are contemplating change, but haven't made the move in the right direction yet. Perhaps your summer clothes are too tight, you saw a picture of yourself in which people were gathering on your shady side, or your doctor made a comment about your size. But instead of taking action, you are caught up in ambivalence, with conflicting feelings of what to do co-habitating your mind. You are wavering, in other words, between the pros and cons of change: "I'd like to be slim, but I don't want to give up my favorite foods." "I know I should exercise, but I don't think I can make the effort."

In thinking about the requirements, you get it that there are benefits to be gained from changing but you are afraid of what you might have to give up in order to change. This mental tug-of-war means you are paralyzed by the high cost of change and stuck in a rut of indecision, not ever attempting to initiate real change. You can't go anywhere while you're straddling a fence.

Yours is also a "haven't gotten around to it yet" or a "put it off 'til next week" attitude, and that's a deal breaker because next week, next month, next year may come, but then again, it may not. It's true, you have substantial challenges, or you wouldn't be reading this book. Ask yourself right now: do you want to continue to be part of this life-wrecking, spirit-breaking epidemic of overweight and obesity? Do you? You must decide once and for all that it is not okay to accept living life as a fence-sitter. Get off the fence and be willing to let yourself want, let yourself reach, let yourself do what you really need to do to solve your weight problem once and for all. It takes courage to change, and it is time for you to claim that courage.

11 to 15: Crossroads

If you answered "yes" to 11 to 15 of these items, you are at the crossroads. That indicates you have been thinking seriously about change for some time now, and perhaps have even made plans to get out of your comfort zone or off the fence. Same-old same-old, going with the flow just doesn't cut it anymore. After conducting some thorough heart-to-heart conversations with yourself, you realize that you are tired of your former wanderings, chasing after the latest, greatest quick-fix diet to come along. You have made a major shift from contemplating change to committing to it. Put another way, you recognize that it is time to begin translating your insights, understandings, and awareness into purposeful, meaningful, constructive action. Equally significant, you believe you can do it.

But don't plan and prepare yourself to death. Life rewards action—a supremely important law of life—not intention, not insight, not understanding. As the old saying goes, "You can't make a hit with the bat on your shoulder." There comes a time when you have to swing that bat. To have what you want, you have to do what it takes. That time is now.

16 to 20: Zero Hour

"Zero hour" is that crucial moment when there is no turning back, and it confronts you to the very core of your self-respect. You have become so sick of your habits and your pattern of living that you realize you can no longer live your life in that way. It's what alcoholics call "hitting rock bottom," or what others call "reaching the end of my rope." It's when you make your mind up that it's not too late, that you deserve more, and that you will deny yourself no longer. It's when you wipe the slate clean and are ready to start over. It's when you decide to reclaim your health and your life. This means that being overweight has taken on a special standing and urgency, lifting high above your other concerns in life. You have boldly said to yourself: "That's enough. I don't care how much it hurts to change. I don't care what I have to give up. I won't take this another second, another minute, another day of my life. I am ready." You know that your dignity and indeed your very being can take only so much, and when you reach this point, you are ready to start living strategically. You want more so you are ready to do more, and are already taking action to get it. Your old way of living is thrown off like a dirty shirt. Change will happen because you make it happen. It will happen because you know what you want and will move toward it in a committed, focused manner.

EXPECT SUCCESS

No matter where you ended up on this readiness continuum, no matter how much you weigh, no matter how disgusted you are with what you see in the mirror, now is your chance, using the seven keys to permanent weight loss, to fix your weight problem for good and live out your best qualities. Believe me when I tell you that it is possible, you can do it, and you are worth it. You are a person with strength, gifts, and talents, capable of achieving your greatest goals. It's like that old saying, "God don't make no junk." You have what it takes to lose weight, be healthy, and live the life you desire and deserve. Now is the time to do it. Now is the time to unlock the doors to permanent weight loss.

Part Two

THE 7 KEYS TO PERMANENT WEIGHT LOSS

4

Key One:
Right Thinking
Unlock the Door to Self-Control

For as he thinks within himself, so is he.
—KING SOLOMON

KEY #1: RIGHT THINKING.

Change your thinking to change your weight. Get rid of self-defeating thought patterns, believe that you will succeed, and you will have mastered the first key necessary to overcome your struggles with your weight. As you begin to think differently, you will succeed and you will maximize your life. What is true about you in your mind, you will live.

As I told you in Chapter 1, everyone—including you—has what I call a "personal truth." This is whatever you, at the absolute core of your being, believe to be true about yourself. It is the story you live, the story you tell yourself about everything that is going on in your life, and this includes your weight and your ability (or lack of ability) to keep your weight in check. You hold powerful beliefs about yourself and these influence you, good or bad, and affect how you approach your weight. Everything you do and feel, and more importantly, how you do it and feel it stems from your personal truth.

You don't have to look far to find negative examples of personal truths that can jump out and ambush your weight-management efforts: you start a weight loss or exercise program to change your shape, but your efforts bite the dust again and again, because you tell yourself that you are a hopeless case who will never succeed. Your personal truth is that of a failure—and honestly, why wouldn't it be?

You have a long history of failure in this arena of weight control, one that you have internalized, and now it dictates to you what your outcome will be.

Yours may be a positive, accurate truth in which you see yourself as healthy and not at all obsessed with your weight, or it may be a real smashup of misbeliefs grounded in your history of failed attempts at weight control. But whatever it is, you have and live your own personal truth, whether you want to or not. Every success or failure you will have flows from that self-determined personal truth. Even if your personal truth is riddled with self-doubt and self-recrimination and self-flagellation, you will live that truth as you go out into the world.

It should be obvious then, why your personal truth is so important. What you believe about yourself, what you treat as your own reality, is dramatically important because it guides and directs your weight-management efforts. So this personal truth business is a big deal, a huge deal. If you don't get yours straight, you are doomed, and even the best-laid plans to get your weight under lasting control will be ruined.

There are very specific processes that go on inside you—internal factors that encompass the things you tell yourself, the things you believe, and the internal dialogue that shapes your behavior. These internal factors comprise the content of your personal truth, and we will examine them here. As we move forward with this key, I intend to show you what your personal truth is, and how it has infiltrated virtually every aspect of your weight control efforts, and that by ridding your personal truth of distortions and self-deception, you can stop living with a backward focus and reconstruct your personal truth in a way to ensure your success in achieving permanent weight loss. I am not going to give you a new personal truth; what you need is already there! It has always been there; it just needs to be cleaned up and rid of all the junk and misinformation you have internalized for too many years.

The first important change, if you are ever to have what you want in terms of your weight, has to happen in your personal truth. That is why we are starting with this key. Let this key serve as your map, your guide, for sorting out the fictional crap from the authentic truth so that you can reject it and finally uncover and live consistently with who you truly are. As you will discover, you have within you everything you will ever need to be, do, and have, anything and everything you will ever want and need.

To help you fully grasp the importance of changing and refining yourself from within, allow me to share with you a story from my family life. When my two sons, Jay and Jordan, were younger, my wife Robin and I would give them birthday parties, as parents ordinarily do, and invite their neighborhood friends over for ice cream and birthday cake. Very early on, we established a tradition for the boys' birthday parties that I would dress up as a clown—clown makeup, red-bulb nose, clown suit, the works (some people say I don't need the costume, but hey, that's beside the point)—and be the entertainment. The kids always loved it and had a ball, squeezing my clown nose and tugging on my raggy clown hair. As part of my act, I carried around with me a huge array of colorful, helium-filled balloons, one for every child to play with at the party.

On one particular occasion, I remember a boy to whom I gave a balloon. Unlike the other little guys who territorially clutched the strings of their balloons, this fella looked up at me and asked, "If I let go of my balloon, will it go up real high?" Moved by his question, I knelt down and responded, "Sure it will, son. It's what's inside your balloon that makes it go up real high."

Isn't this exactly the truth about us? Our inner thoughts, beliefs, self-perceptions, and emotions can give us a lift for a positive outcome, or hold us back in complete inertia. You may be telling yourself that you will never lose weight, or that it is too hard, or that you have no self-control. If you accept these thoughts as your personal truth, you will only sabotage your efforts to manage your weight. Your negative thoughts and beliefs will hold you back. And because these internal messages create your emotional state, what you tell yourself can make you feel stressed, anxious, worried, depressed—and more apt to binge or overeat. You mustn't be duped by your own self-talk, any more than if someone else told you that you can't lose weight or get your life under control.

Unless you eliminate self-defeating thoughts, they will actually gain momentum, becoming more deeply lodged in the habitual patterns of your life and more unyielding to change. Of course, before we rid you of these thoughts, we must identify and acknowledge them, and we will do that in this key with a series of invaluable audits that will give you the clarity you need to make important changes in your thoughts, attitudes, and beliefs.

If you have ever been to a circus, perhaps you have seen six-ton elephants tethered by rope to little wooden stakes. Have you ever wondered why one of these powerful animals doesn't yank that stake out of the ground and stampede off? When the elephants are young and powerless, they are attached by heavy chains to immovable steel stakes. The baby elephants tug and pull, but no matter how hard they try, the chains will not break and the stakes will not come out of the ground. As the elephants grow and get stronger, they come to believe that they cannot move anywhere as long as there is a stake in the ground nearby, no matter how tiny or weak the stake. They don't try to break loose because they think they can't.

So it is with people. If you are like those circus elephants, you've allowed your thoughts and actions to limit you, and like those elephants, you may not have been aware that you had choices. Well, you may not have been aware before, but I'm telling you now that you do have choices, you do have power; now you know. You don't have to stay mindlessly tied to stakes of wrong thinking and self-destructive behavior. You can "pull up the stakes," transcend your conditioning, and reprogram yourself for success rather than failure.

There are many experts who believe that obesity is a disease of choice, and I agree. There are not many diseases of choice, but obesity is certainly one of them. If you gain weight, you are choosing behaviors that encourage the development of obesity, setting up a lifestyle geared toward being overweight. Some of you are fat because you want to be that way, and you are feeding a need, or any number of needs. For others of you, obesity is a disease of metabolism; you may not necessarily eat more than slender people do, and you may indeed exercise, but for biochemical reasons, your body burns food less efficiently. Even if you are in this group, there are choices you can make to manage metabolic and biochemical logjams, and I will talk to you about them in Chapter 11.

How you approach this issue of choice is absolutely critical to your success. You are creating the situation and the state of health you are in. Once you wake up to this fact, you can begin to see, hopefully with crystal-clear definition what choices you have made that led to this result. Then you can start changing thoughts, attitudes, behaviors, and choices to get a different result.

That is not all bad news. Accepting your role in your weight problem, acknowledging that you are accountable, means that you get it. It means that you understand that the solutions lie within you. This gives you a tremendous head start toward permanent weight loss.

With this key, you will learn how to change your internal dialogue and, in doing so, regain self-control and peace of mind. When you begin to think, feel, and behave differently, when you are on the right track internally and emotionally, you'll quickly discover that, like that released balloon I described above, there is an enormous energy that uplifts you.

I realize that when I start talking about mental activity, your understandable reaction may be, "He's asking me to examine my thinking and deal with my emotions. I don't care about that junk. That's just something shrinks talk about. I just don't think about myself that much."

Trust me, I'm not going to spout a bunch of "guru-ized" stuff about thoughts and emotions, or tell you to go up on a mountaintop and get in touch with your "inner child." What I am going to give you is an unbelievably practical set of tools, techniques, and exercises so that you can observe, evaluate, and challenge what has been sabotaging your weight-control efforts internally. Please don't underestimate or discard what I'm talking about here. Once you take control of your internal activity, you're going to be amazed at the power you have to get your weight under control. Losing weight and keeping it off is not just about food. If all you did was change what you eat, you'd lose some weight, but you would not keep if off for very long because you would not have redefined your life from the inside out. For you to achieve permanent weight loss, change must come totally from within you. This is where the real power to create lasting results is found, and what you are about to do here will give you that power.

INTERNAL AUDITS

Because you cannot change what you do not acknowledge, we will begin unlocking this door with two internal audits, designed to help you clarify thought patterns that may be holding you back. The first of these audits will look into your *weight locus of control* (WLOC), a particular mind-set that reveals who or what you credit or blame for the shape you're in. Some people, for example, blame their obesity on their genes, their metabolism, or on their food-pushing relatives. Some use the excuse that they just can't diet because their husband or children would suffer if they didn't have cookies, chips, or other foods around the house as snacks. Others believe that the power to lose weight and stay fit resides solely within themselves. And some people have a fatalistic mind-set toward their weight gain—the "it's just my bad luck" attitude.

Identifying your primary weight locus of control is important, because once you know what it is, you can exercise greater control over your thinking, feelings, and behavior. You'll be awakened to powerful resources at your disposal—resources that can help you finally achieve your weight loss goals. You'll be able to stop destructive behavior such as overeating, bingeing, on-again, off-again dieting. And you'll have a new measure of self-control over your mind and body.

With this in mind, let's complete the short questionnaire to determine your WLOC. Please be very honest in your answers. It's probably easy for you to ascertain what might be a desirable answer, but that won't help you. Nothing short of complete unvarnished truth and candor will be of any use to you here.

Once you have finished the questionnaire, we'll analyze your score, to better understand your approach to weight control, and consider ways to begin changing specific elements of your locus that are flowing in a negative direction.

YOUR WEIGHT LOCUS OF CONTROL

For each statement below, decide how much you agree or disagree with it. Of the four answer choices, select the one that best expresses how you feel about the statement: if you agree totally without reservations, then circle "a" agree; "b" if you agree slightly; "c" if you disagree slightly; or "d" if you disagree completely.

Part A. Internal Weight Locus of Control

1. Gaining, losing, and maintaining weight is entirely up to me.
   a. Agree.
   b. Agree slightly.
   c. Disagree slightly.
   d. Disagree.

2. I am overweight as a result of my eating habits.
   a. Agree.
   b. Agree slightly.
   c. Disagree slightly.
   d. Disagree.

3. I am overweight as a result of being inactive or not getting enough exercise.
   a. Agree.
   b. Agree slightly.
   c. Disagree slightly.
   d. Disagree.

4. If I set realistic, measurable goals, I can lose weight no matter what.
   a. Agree.
   b. Agree slightly.
   c. Disagree slightly.
   d. Disagree.

5. Failure to keep my weight off is due to poor effort on my part.
   a. Agree.
   b. Agree slightly.
   c. Disagree slightly.
   d. Disagree.

Part B. External Weight Locus of Control

6. Family history has most determined my weight and size.
   a. Agree.
   b. Agree slightly.

    c. Disagree slightly.
    d. Disagree.

7. I need a structured, formal diet program, or else I have difficulty losing weight.
    a. Agree.
    b. Agree slightly.
    c. Disagree slightly.
    d. Disagree.

8. I depend on good doctors or nutritionists to help me lose weight.
    a. Agree.
    b. Agree slightly.
    c. Disagree slightly.
    d. Disagree.

9. I need prescription diet pills or other diet aids to lose weight.
    a. Agree.
    b. Agree slightly.
    c. Disagree slightly.
    d. Disagree.

10. I overeat because there is too much tempting food in my environment.
    a. Agree.
    b. Agree slightly.
    c. Disagree slightly.
    d. Disagree.

Part C. Chance Weight Locus of Control

11. Being at my ideal weight is a matter of good fortune.
    a. Agree.
    b. Agree slightly.
    c. Disagree slightly.
    d. Disagree.

12. My failure to lose weight is just bad luck.
    a. Agree.
    b. Agree slightly.

c. Disagree slightly.

d. Disagree.

13. I will go off my diet if I have a bad day.
    a. Agree.
    b. Agree slightly.
    c. Disagree slightly.
    d. Disagree.

14. No matter if I gain weight, lose weight, or stay the same, it is just going to happen, and that's life.
    a. Agree.
    b. Agree slightly.
    c. Disagree slightly.
    d. Disagree.

15. I am very lucky if I stick to my exercise program.
    a. Agree.
    b. Agree slightly.
    c. Disagree slightly.
    d. Disagree.

SCORING

You will score yourself separately for each of the three parts of the WLOC assessment (Internal, External, and Chance). For each "Agree" answer, give yourself 4 points; for each "Agree slightly" answer, give yourself 3 points; for each "Disagree slightly" answer, give yourself 2 points; and for each "Disagree" answer, give yourself 1 point. Record your totals in the spaces below:

Part A. Internal _____

Part B. External _____

Part C. Chance _____

Your responses to the questions for each part of the assessment generated three separate scores, each ranging from five to twenty. For each of the three parts of the test—Internal, External, and Chance—your scores place you into one of four categories: very low, low, average, or high for each of the three parts of the test, in accordance with the following chart:

Part A: Internal Weight Locus of Control

5 to 7: Very low attribution of your weight to internal responsibilities

8 to 11: Low attribution of your weight to internal responsibilities

12 to 16: Average attribution of your weight to internal responsibilities

17 to 20: High attribution of your weight to internal responsibilities

Part B: External Weight Locus of Control

5 to 7: Very low attribution of your weight to external responsibilities

8 to 11: Low attribution of your weight to external responsibilities

12 to 16: Average attribution of your weight to external responsibilities

17 to 20: High attribution of your weight to external responsibilities

Part C: Chance Weight Locus of Control

5 to 7: Very low attribution of your weight to chance

8 to 11: Low attribution of your weight to chance

12 to 16: Average attribution of your weight to chance

17 to 20: High attribution of your weight to chance

Internal WLOC

If you are in the average to high end of internal WLOC (12 to 20), you have an *internal weight locus of control*. This means that you operate from a position that says, "If I don't lose weight, it's my fault. If I lose weight, it's because of my efforts." You feel you have a direct bearing on your results, through your own actions, interactions, traits, and characteristics, and you accept responsibility, as well as credit, for how things turn out. If you're overweight, for example, you'll admit that you got that way because you did not eat right or did not exercise enough. You tend to take the majority of accountability for correcting your condition, including making lifestyle changes, and you hold yourself responsible for change in your life. These are positive attributes.

Advice: be aware, though, that there are downsides to having an internal orientation. For example, you might find it difficult to seek counsel from other people or to consult external sources of information for help. Ignoring external resources at your disposal cuts you off from beneficial insights, guidance, and support from knowledgeable people such as physicians, nutritionists, and other healthcare providers.

If your thinking is too internally controlled, your locus of control can create another problem for you. You may tend to internalize your failures and dwell on them. When you engage in this type of thinking, then you have a running internal dialogue with yourself that is negative, one that puts yourself down, engages in "mountain-out-of-molehill thinking," and convinces yourself that your limitations are too great for lasting success to be realized. And when you think along these lines, you're discounting your own abilities and extinguishing your goals of ever controlling your weight. You must work on how you interpret your failures, become aware of your negative internal dialogue, and work to change it. This key will help you.

Recognize too that there will be events over which you have no control. For example, you are not to blame for missing your morning walk because there's a real gully-washer outside. If you say, "I'm mad at myself because I didn't get to walk today," you are inappropriately internalizing. You're blaming yourself for the weather!

Or suppose you've had a perfectly compliant, motivated week. You've eaten nutritiously, and you exercised according to schedule. But the scale says otherwise. Getting mad at yourself would be a mistake, since other factors may be responsible, such as water retention, the addition of muscle to your body because you're exercising (muscle weighs more than fat), or the fact that your body has reached a plateau and is adjusting accordingly. So be realistic about what you can control and what you can't. Pay attention to how good you feel, or how loose your clothes are. These are the hallmarks of real progress.

External WLOC

A high or average score on the external scale (12 to 20) implies an *external weight locus of control*, characterized by highly dependent reliance on powerful others or powerful influences for your success or failure at losing weight. Let me give you an example of how external thinking might manifest in your own life. Think back to one of those times when you went on a diet, you lost a lot of weight, and your friends, with their oohs and ahhs, asked you how you did it. Because you tend to be externally oriented, you probably replied by telling them it was the Such and Such Diet. You credited a diet, instead of your own self-determination, for your success. With this orientation style, you believe that credit for your good results rests outside yourself, on someone or something else. Maybe it is the latest, greatest new diet. Maybe it is a nutritionist or a doctor with whom you worked. Maybe it is a prescription diet drug or a surgical procedure such as a gastric bypass that you credit for your weight loss. When you succeed, you take little or no ownership of this positive outcome.

By the same token, when you fail to lose weight, cycle back up, or bomb out altogether, you take little or no ownership of that, either. You blame being overweight on any number of factors other than the quart of Rocky Road ice cream you have enjoyed every night for the past five years. You feel your weight has nothing to do with your own choices to overeat or binge. It always has to do with other people, other things, and other situations, never with your own actions. For example, you might say you regained all your weight because a particular diet "stopped working" for you. Or maybe you're like the middle-aged lug who still wants to eat the way he ate in high school—burgers, fries, pizza, beer, and so on—and still expects to weigh what he weighed way back then. He says that his metabolism is too slow. He never thinks for a moment that he's sporting a spare tire because, like some people, he may be too lazy to exercise anymore.

No matter what the situation or circumstance, you assign blame elsewhere—even if the fault is yours and not something or someone else's.

Advice: if you persist in thinking that your weight is controlled entirely by external forces, you'll have a difficult time losing unwanted pounds. By pinning the blame on your family, your genes, a metabolism problem, or a diet that "didn't work," you may be misdiagnosing the reasons behind your weight problem. When you misdiagnose, that means you will mistreat it too, and fail to do what is actually and realistically called for.

This can ruin your chances of permanent weight loss and control because you're not taking ownership of what's truly your fault. You're not facing up to the fact that your poor eating habits and lack of exercise have made you fat. Give yourself a reality check here; there are enough things that affect your weight for which you are clearly and undeniably responsible.

Your solution is to move your locus of control from the external to the internal. In doing so, you make yourself responsible for your own choices and actions. When you begin to see that your particular weight struggles may have little to do with anything outside yourself, your power to change is enormous.

Another huge problem with being in the external niche is that you tend to leapfrog from diet to diet in an elusive pursuit of the "one that works" and because that doesn't exist, you get frustrated and you get defeated—and as a result you soon find yourself behaving your way back to Blobsville. Your weight-control attempts are characterized by on-again, off-again dieting. When this happens, you will just keep spinning your wheels and staying stuck in the same old ruts.

With too much externally-directed thinking, you'll set goals for yourself that are too low, or not set any goals at all. For example, you might tell yourself, "I can't achieve my ideal weight. Something will stand in my way." This is all negative externalizing behavior. Imagine the consequences that flow from that type of thinking. Whenever you try to lose weight, you've given up your self-control and crushed whatever personal resolve you might have had. Quit thinking like that, and start recognizing that you actively influence positive events in your life. Start pedaling on your own personal power.

Chance WLOC

If you are in the average to high end (12 to 20), you have a *chance weight locus of control*. You are basically telling yourself that you have little or no belief in yourself or anything else. You may not see any point in changing your diet, starting an exercise program, or taking any personal responsibility for your health because you believe that your behavior has nothing to do with your choices. If you're fat or otherwise unhealthy, or even if you lose some weight, it's an accidental occurrence, a roll of the dice in the game of chance. In your perceptual set, every result, every outcome is due to fate, accident, or just plain luck.

Make no mistake: this mind-set of chance has nothing to do with self-discipline. It's different from not wanting to change your habits just because you don't want to discipline yourself. Chance is a feeling of powerlessness: you don't see the point of discipline and therefore have no motivation to change.

Advice: while research indicates that people with internal and external WLOC will lose weight, high-chance people have less hope of success. That's because they believe that there's no point in even trying to change because neither they nor anyone else has any input to or control over their lives.

Dominated by the mind-set of chance, they think people should love them no matter what they look like. After all, it's just that they were dealt a bad hand. If this is your profile, you are probably treating yourself and your health very poorly. When you live like this, with so little regard for yourself, you are cheating not just yourself, but also everyone around you.

If your internal viewpoint is, "What difference does it make anyway?" or "If fortune goes my way, it'll happen," then you're likely to spend the rest of your life in an overweight and unhealthy condition.

You are missing out on critical opportunities to make a difference in your own life and health.

I trust that at this point you've begun to recognize that your weight locus of control contains lies and faulty logic that form at the core of your personal truth, and that you must start nudging yourself in some different directions. Maybe your thinking needs to become less internally oriented, less externally oriented, or moved off the chance orientation altogether. This will require that you start questioning whether you're appropriately "giving credit where credit is due," that you begin living with more self-determination in certain areas, and that you become more involved in governing the outcomes in your life.

INTERNAL DIALOGUE AUDIT

Your belief about what or who is in control of your weight and your health strongly influences your internal dialogue or self-talk—the private inner conversation you have with yourself about everything that is going on in your life. It involves the negatives you fixate on; self-criticisms such as guilt and shame; and the self-deceptions and distorted views that invade your life. If your internal dialogue is negative and self-condemning, you're creating obstacles for yourself that you don't need, and you can miss real opportunities for success in truly managing your weight.

In this next important audit, I'd like you to tune in to your self-talk in order to identify exactly what it is that you tell yourself. Write down what you say to yourself about these topics:

- Your appearance

- Your body shape

- Your ability to manage your weight

- Your exercise level

- Your self-control

- Your general health

Next, look back over your writing. How would you describe the overall tone or mood of your self-talk? Is it positive, upbeat? Or is it pessimistic, defeatist, or self-condemning? Underline any writing that you think illustrates either especially positive or especially negative self-talk.

Also, what does your writing tell you about your weight locus of control? Does it add any new insight? Is your self-talk oriented externally, internally, or in accordance with chance? Record your answer.

Don't toss your important reflection in the trash can. Hang on to it, because you'll need to refer to it later. It contains some valuable information that will help you understand your personal content with greater clarity than ever before.

MAXIMIZE YOUR WEIGHT LOSS THROUGH SELF-TALK

Throughout your day, you're engaged in dialogues with many other people, but your most active and consistent dialogue is the conversation you have with yourself. You may be with ten different people throughout any given day, but you're with yourself day in and day out, and you talk to yourself more than everybody else in your life combined.

Your self-talk is the real-time mental conversation, the flow of thoughts, that you have with yourself about everything that is going on in your life. It is what you are saying to yourself, about yourself, about the world, about what happens to you, right now, all the time.

Your thoughts are behavior too. Choosing thoughts contributes to your experiences, because when you choose your thoughts, you choose the consequences that are associated with those thoughts. If you choose thoughts that are self-negating and demeaning, for example, then you choose the consequences of low self-esteem and low self-confidence that flow from those thoughts. If you choose thoughts contaminated with sadness, then you will create an experience of depression that flows from those thoughts.

And we can't discuss consequences without mentioning the physiological consequences of our thinking. When you choose your thoughts, you also choose the physiological outcomes that are associated with those thoughts. For every thought you have, a physiological event occurs in unison with that thought. Take anger, for example. An angry reaction can produce elevated blood pressure, increased heart rate, skin rashes, and other harmful physiological events.

Here's another example, one that's closer to our topic of weight management: imagine thinking, "I really don't like exercise." Your body reacts to this depressed thought by suppressing energy and action. Your body has conformed to that central computer message. With such negative internal programming, is it any wonder that your performance is poor, or that you can't stick to an exercise program for very long? Or perhaps your self-talk is filled with sour-note messages like "I'll never lose weight" or "I hate the way I look in the mirror." Those thoughts will work against you; just count on it.

What's more, since thoughts are behaviors, you must be alert to what payoffs, or rewards, you are getting from the things you tell yourself. At some level, your self-talk is working for you. For example: if you tell yourself, "I don't have time to exercise," then you're giving yourself an easy out for not ever trying to become more active. There's your payoff: you have an excuse for not doing anything about your activity level, and you avoid the pressure of reaching for something better.

Bottom line: your thoughts powerfully program you. That's why our focus with this key will be to jettison any negative self-talk you're dragging around with you and replace it with positive, productive internal dialogue.

But please don't confuse this with "think yourself thin." I don't believe something as important as weight control can be summed up in such a pat phrase, and I'm not here to tell you that the answer to your weight problem is to think good thoughts all the time. If you try to "think thin," I guarantee you, you'll stay as spread out as cold supper. This is about looking analytically at your internal dialogue, blowing the whistle on it, and changing interactions that are in direct opposition to your weight loss goals. The steps you are about to take, right here, will give you the added momentum and power to be healthy and fit for the rest of your life.

STEP ONE: BECOME AWARE OF YOUR FAULTY THINKING

Typically, faulty thinking, especially about weight and weight control, runs along predictable lines. In my work with overweight patients, I have identified ten of the most common self-defeating messages that can undermine a person's weight-control efforts. Obviously, if you know what these messages are and become aware of them in your own life, you can change the course of your weight-control efforts. The ten most common self-defeating messages I have identified are:

1. Externalizing/Internalizing

Your weight locus of control, which we looked at earlier, orchestrates and guides the content of your self-talk. If you tend to be externally oriented, for example, a lot of your internal dialogue might sound like, "I can't lose weight on my own. I'll have to take a diet drug." Or if you have an internal WLOC, you might be telling yourself, "If I'm going to achieve my goals, I've got to work out harder each time." With a chance WLOC, you might tell yourself, "Being overweight is just in the cards. There's nothing I can do about it."

Whatever primary locus is at work in your life, it tends to be an influential force on what you say to yourself. Too much thinking in any one of these three dynamics—internal, external, or chance—can create outcomes you don't want. Thus, if you've acknowledged that you're inappropriately internalizing, externalizing, or being too fatalistic (chance), then you must stop letting yourself be pushed and pulled by that dynamic. Realistically assess what you can control and what you cannot, and take action to make a difference in your life.

2. Labeling

Labels are self-descriptions in your internal dialogue that reflect certain conclusions you've reached about yourself. Many of these labels came from within you when you observed yourself messing up in life, or they have come from other people. Maybe you have been ridiculed all your life for your weight, or have been the brunt of cruel fat jokes.

In America, if you are overweight, you are stereotyped with labels such as "lazy," "sloppy," and "ugly." That's not fair, nor is it legal in certain employment situations, but it is a grievous part of life if you are overweight. People are going to be insensitive and treat you badly. Fair or unfair, it's the way things are.

But whatever their source, you tend to internalize these labels, believe your labels, and live by your labels. They can become the definition of yourself if you let them. People dealing with weight problems typically label themselves as "failures" when they can't lose weight. Once you accept such a label as valid, you annihilate your self-confidence, your self-determination, and your longing for a healthier, more ideal weight. If you believe a negative label, then you'll absolutely miss evidence to the contrary.

3. Frustration Thinking

Many of you, when faced with going on a diet or starting an exercise program, tell yourself that you cannot tolerate the frustration and discomfort of not eating your favorite foods or having to haul your ample rear to the gym. Unable to stand the discomfort of changing, you have a low frustration set, expressed in thinking that goes something like this, "It's too hard. It's easier to stay fat. I can't be bothered with exercise."

So to protect yourself, you convince yourself that any type of dietary or lifestyle change is just too difficult. This type of internal dialogue is marked by constant pessimism, and you upset yourself with these limiting thoughts. One reason you persist in it is its payoff: you're avoiding frustration and discomfort. But in doing so, you're cluttering up your mind with all kinds of BS, so every time you think about losing weight, you quit before you even get to the starting line.

4. Fortune-Telling

Like an internal psychic, your self-talk makes predictions about your performance, and when negative, this prediction tends to be a doom-and-gloom type prophecy. Your internal fortune-telling might run the gamut from "This won't work; I'll never lose weight; I will fail; I've got too much to lose" to "I'll never drop those last five or ten pounds." When this type of internal dialogue is really active, rationally confident thoughts get shunted out of your mind because they aren't as dominant or demanding. In essence, this negative internal dialogue can become a vicious cycle of self-fulfilling prophecy, controlling your thinking and predicting the outcome you will have.

The smashing of the four-minute mile barrier in 1954 is a classic example of a self-fulfilling prophecy. People all over the world believed that running this distance in under four minutes was physiologically impossible for any human being, and so it never happened, until a young physician named Roger Bannister believed he could do it. And he did. In his legendary, record-breaking race, Bannister sprinted across the finish line in a time of three minutes and fifty-nine point four seconds. But what is truly instructive about this story is that in the very next year, twelve more runners broke this previously unsurpassable mark, and today athletes do it all the time.

If you're working at managing your weight, tune in to whether you are making predictions about your performance. If you are, you could be setting yourself up for an outcome you don't want.

5. All-or-Nothing Thinking

Suppose you step on the scales after you get out of the shower and the news is not good. If your internal dialogue tells you, "I gained weight again. All my attempts are useless," you're engaging in all-or-nothing thinking. You're saying to yourself that the situations, circumstances, events, and results in your life are all good or all bad, black or white, with no shades of gray in between. That dialogue, with all of its self-defeating messages, is particularly damaging because it can reactivate unwanted behavior.

Look at it this way: you have dinner one night with your family and decide to have a small piece of pie for dessert—that's fine, but then your internal dialogue kicks in, and you say, "What the heck, I've blown my diet. I might as well eat the whole pie." With an all-or-nothing conversation with yourself, you entertain thoughts that because you ate a piece of pie, all was lost, so you might as well go from a bite to a full-blown binge. It is this type of distorted self-talk that often precedes addictive relapses among alcoholics, drug addicts—and overeaters.

6. Catastrophizing

When you evaluate events, do you exaggerate their meaning or significance? For example, does your internal dialogue ever chatter along these lines: "If I don't lose weight this time, I'll never do it." "I gained two pounds. This is horrible." "My boyfriend will hate me if I gain weight." If your internal dialogue sounds like this, you are catastrophizing—expecting the worst or making a melodrama out of everything that happens to you. For you, none of life's events, even the everyday ones, are ordinary. Every pound you gain is the most you've ever gained. Every slipup you have or mistake you make is a disaster. Every comment made to you is the rudest or most devastating you've ever heard. Like all forms of negative self-talk, this internal dialogue is self-defeating because you are reacting illogically toward a situation instead of viewing it rationally. When you talk to yourself like this, it can lead to a loss of self-control over healthy behavior.

7. Pipe Dreaming

Maybe thoughts of wanting to look like a fashion model or a Hollywood hunk are passing through your mind. Your internal dialogue is daring you to entertain fantasies of having the perfect body. Or maybe what you hear is a message that you can drop two sizes in two weeks. On the surface, this kind of talk may sound like positive, "I believe in myself" dialogue, but in truth it is very negative because the messages are unreasonable and unrealistic. Imposing unattainable goals on yourself leads to feelings of failure because these dreams do not materialize. If you're chasing after impossible pipe dreams, you're bound to be disappointed. You have to get real about what you can really achieve.

8. Gut-Level Reasoning

Sometimes the toxic inner environment that your internal dialogue sets up stems from transient, unreliable feelings that you may experience at any given time. For example, the belief that "I feel fat" gets translated by your internal dialogue into "I must look fat." You accept a feeling as absolute truth, and once you begin believing it, why would you continue to process data to the contrary? You might have a heap of evidence that runs counter to your looking fat, but your data-processing ability is so out of whack that you don't see or hear the more accurate, reliable information.

9. Self-Downing

When you come down on yourself, your internal dialogue cranks up its volume, becoming so loud that it crowds out other, more relevant and truthful information. If you're depressed about your weight, for example, your internal dialogue is likely to scream out put-downs such as, "I can't lose weight. I don't have any self-control." You start condemning yourself for not succeeding, or obsessing about what you didn't do or could have done better. I'm sure you've said these things to yourself thousands of times. The problem is, if you treat this internal browbeating as gospel truth, it becomes reality for you.

Understand that much of this dialogue, in which you put yourself down so persistently and destructively, has been told to you by others in your life. It may be that your parents, partner, or relatives have verbally assaulted you with remarks like "You can't get thin," "You don't have what it takes to lose weight or be attractive," or "You'll always be as big as a house." Their words have gotten inside your head, poisoning your thoughts and distorting how you see yourself, and have been a major determinant of your internal dialogue. But hear me out on this: it's bad enough if people in your life put you down, but it becomes disastrous if you internalize their put-downs, take over for them, and wind up kicking your own butt. You've got to acknowledge that this may be happening in your own mind, and blow the whistle on it. Only then will you have the power to change these highly destructive internal responses.

10. Poor Me Thinking

Another particularly treacherous form of self-downing is "poor me thinking," born out of feeling deprived or out of the fear of getting hungry. It can surface when you go on a diet that is overly restrictive. You find it hard to envision ever being able to enjoy a party, go on vacation, eat what other people are eating, and so forth. This is a conversation in which you start feeling sorry for yourself, and a lot of your self-talk might sound like: "It's not fair that other people can eat cream puffs all day, and I can't." "I hate depriving myself of one of life's pleasures." "I shouldn't have to work this hard to get in shape. It's easier for other people to do it." "I'll get too hungry." "I can't go to any parties."

What can take this self-talk (or any self-talk, for that matter) from a whisper to a whoop is poor nutrition. If you're indeed following a diet with limited choices, this can alter your mental state for the worse. Poor nutrition throws your physiological balance off just enough to create a depressed mood, and with it, its underlying negative self-talk.

The end point of this type of thinking is highly destructive. For example, you may overeat or binge in order to compensate for your feelings of deprivation. Feeling sorry for yourself, you embark on a feeding frenzy in an attempt to cope. But what you fail to rationally take into account is that you can still go to parties, you can still go on vacations, and you can still do anything you want to do. You just need to focus on the camaraderie, the scenery, the activities, and the "battery recharge" you get from relaxation and recreation, rather than center every occasion on food. Think about deprivation another way: by overeating, you're depriving yourself of a healthy weight, an attractive appearance, self-regard, and peace of mind.

These are some classic types of internal dialogue that may be sabotaging you. I hope you've recognized from this discussion that internal dialogue, when negative, is relentless, and can be highly destructive. If you're demeaning yourself, your body, and your personal control, and your internal dialogue shows it, you'll be compromised. Everybody criticizes their bodies. Everybody has self-doubt. Everybody has anxiety. But when any of these kinds of messages get their hooks in you, when they infiltrate your thinking, it becomes more difficult to get closer to what you really want to have and do. If you passively accept the messages of your internal dialogue, if you let it speak to you unchallenged, you have just stonewalled your chances of getting your weight under lasting control.

STEP TWO: CHALLENGE YOUR FAULTY THINKING

If your weight-control problems are due at least in part to errors in your thinking, to faulty assumptions about what is going on in your life, you have to work to challenge that thinking. Like a prosecutor in a courtroom, you must put your thoughts on the witness stand, take a hard look at the evidence and the testimony, and confront them with facts, truth, and realities.

Toward that end, you must ask four questions. These are questions that I've talked about in prior books, and I emphasize them here because they have come to be a personal yardstick for me in my life in order to make sure that my internal dialogue is rational and productive. These questions can help pave the way to positive and empowering thoughts in your own life. This stuff works for me, and I know it will work powerfully for you in your weight-control efforts. Once you get used to testing every thought and perception against these questions, you'll get to the point that trying to slip a lie past you will be like trying to bag flies. Here are the four questions:

Is your internal dialogue true?

Most of us don't question the truthfulness of our internal dialogue; instead we infect it with many of the self-defeating messages I just described for you. Take Dan, for example, a former patient of mine who frequently lapsed into eating junk food when by himself. His self-talk screamed, "I can't help bingeing when I'm alone." What I asked him went like this: "Is that really true? Is there nothing else, nothing at all that you can do when you are alone? Isn't there some activity, something that doesn't involve food, that you could do rather than binge?" Once we examined the evidence concerning the situation, Dan started generating a practically endless list of activities he could do instead of bingeing.

Start reacting to your internal responses as if they were statements on a true-false quiz (I used to love that kind of test back in school because there was at least a 50 percent chance I'd get the right answer!). Are your responses true or are they false? Can you prove it? For example, what is the evidence that you are a failure? Is this just something that you believe now because your mother or father told you that you'd always be fat and you internalized this message because you believed them and accepted it as true, without deliberately testing it? Where's exhibit A, B, or C that you are a failure? Surely, you've had numerous successes in your life so maybe this is not true at all. Maybe you've never really thought about it. If you don't evaluate your thinking and sort out what's true and what's false, then you'll act on something that you simply accept as true, perhaps mindlessly, with no consideration of measuring it against a standard of authenticity. You've got to start challenging your internal dialogue in this regard, and expose the fictions and the falsehoods. No matter what you're telling yourself, test everything against this question. Should it be true, then you must deal with it. If it's not true, kick it out!

Does your internal dialogue serve your best interests?

It's a sure bet that you're clinging to certain thoughts and beliefs because they serve as a handy excuse or justification for why you've botched your weight-control efforts in the past. A good example is: "Because obesity runs in my family, I just can't lose weight."

When you hold such views, you're locked in classic victim thinking. You're reacting to the world as a victim, clinging to the belief that your weight problem can't possibly be your fault. You've been conning yourself without cross-examining yourself, because no one's listening to your internal dialogue except you. You've been willing to accept your excuses at face value and you've been letting yourself off far too easily.

But let me ask you this: is holding on to the excuse that you're a victim, blaming others for your results, really going to help you get in shape? Does it bring you happiness, peace, calm, and fulfillment? Is it working for you? If you answered No, No, and No, then stop listening to your own justifications and excuses for why you are putting up with these thoughts and beliefs, actions and inactions, that are not working for you. If it's not working, let go of it!

Bottom line: there are no victims, only volunteers. You are creating the situations you're in; you're creating the thoughts and emotions that flow from those situations. You must embrace the fact that you own your problems and take action to solve them.

Does your internal dialogue advance and protect your health?

Do negative thoughts about exercise make you avoid it and put your health and vitality on the line? For example, does the fact that you've grown buttery prevent you from going to exercise classes because you are too self-conscious about your body, so you just stay home and do nothing? Does your self-imposed disgust over your appearance lead to habitual bingeing on sugary foods and processed foods that exacts a physical toll you can ill afford? Are your reactions to stress generating physical accord in your body? Or are you constantly worked up, wearing down your body and subjecting yourself to disease? It may be that now is the time to understand that holding such beliefs is not helping you; that in fact, they are hurting you.

Is your internal dialogue helping you achieve your weight-management goals?

I can't express it more plainly than this. If your goal is to achieve permanent weight loss, and experience the physical and emotional health that stems from it, then you must test your internal responses against that goal. Given your goals, how does your current thinking help you get there? If you want to look better, feel better, be better, how does repeating "This won't work," or "It's too hard," help you achieve permanent weight control? Are your thoughts, beliefs, and attitudes moving you closer to what you want? Or are they leading you farther and farther away from a normal, healthy weight?

When your internal dialogue isn't true, when it doesn't serve your best interests, when it's hurting your health, when it's standing between you and your efforts to reach your weight loss goals, then it's time for you to jack up your thinking and do something different. It's time to generate positive, healthy internal dialogue that does everything the negative internal crap does not. If you shake up your internal messaging system, challenging in particular those views you hold about yourself, rather than blindly or habitually accepting them as the whole truth and nothing but, then your level of control over your weight will strengthen, and I mean fast.

Step Three: Restructure Your Thinking with Positive Internal Dialogue

You've seen through the examples here that internal dialogue can be highly negative and disruptive. The flip side to this is a positive type of internal dialogue—one that is rationally optimistic and productive.

Now, I am not here to be your Norman Vincent Peale and tell you that the secret to success lies in the "power of positive thinking." That is not at all what I am talking about. Positive, rational internal dialogue differs greatly from the power of positive thinking. Here's what I mean: positive internal dialogue consists of thoughts and messages that are grounded in reality, not lies, assumptions, or opinion. It is truthful engagement with the world that allows you to live in accord with reality.

What positive internal dialogue is not is a bunch of preachy mantras, wrapped up in truth-denying rah-rah affirmations. Let's say for example that you're in the habit of eating a bag of potato chips every day after work, while reciting to yourself, "I'm a good person just like I am." Who's kidding whom here, anyway? The truth is that you're not requiring enough of yourself in terms of self-control. You're putting food away like a boardinghouse cat. This is not even close to what I call positive, healthy internal dialogue. If you tell yourself good things that are not based in reality, this brand of internal dialogue is not at all positive. It all comes back to your personal truth, and you know that is a truth you live. Lie to yourself, and you will pay the price of never really achieving your weight loss goals over the long-term.

A rational, healthy internal dialogue would tell you the truth so you can do something about it. If you've got a problem, admit it. Have an honest conversation with yourself. For example: "I'm not powerless over this behavior. I'm in charge of myself. I have to choose what's more important: reactive overeating or taking care of my health. It's my choice, and I can do something about it." Whatever you're telling yourself, tune in to it, challenge its authenticity, and replace it with fact, not fiction. Don't give yourself rah-rah self-con jobs.

We discussed earlier that negative internal dialogue physiologically suppresses action and energy. When you begin to nurture your mind with rational, healthy thoughts, a similar process occurs, but one that is infinitely more transformative and empowering in its effect. If you are thinking rationally positive thoughts, your body and brain are energized and primed for success. Scientists have been studying this mind-body connection for years, and their research consistently shows that the thoughts we have can maximize performance in nearly every aspect of life. Musicians perform with fewer errors when they hold self-affirming thoughts. Salespeople increase their sales quotas. Athletes increase their speed and accuracy.

The same necessity for changing your internal dialogue applies to you. The thoughts you have about how you are going to execute your weight-control strategies will determine how well you do. That's why you must restructure your thoughts. This involves replacing negative internal dialogue with fact-based messages that drive you to do so much more than just get by.

I want you to root out the self-defeating thinking that holds you back and incorporate rational, balanced, and productive dialogue into your thinking. Doing this means that you must have a new conversation with yourself that responds to negative messages truthfully and positively. The accompanying table provides examples to guide you.

However unhelpful and unhealthy your thought patterns, you must recognize that you no longer need to think like this. You can create an internal dialogue that is healthy, constructive, and joyful. That's what this step will help you do.

It's now time for you to identify what goes through your head, test its validity, and generate positive balancing internal dialogue. You'll accomplish this by completing the chart below. It asks you to do three things:

Record instances of negative self-talk that may be contaminating your thoughts;

Test the validity of those thoughts using the four questions we discussed earlier in this chapter; and

Replace those self-defeating thoughts with positive self-talk (restructuring).

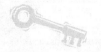

TABLE 2. RIGHT THINKING RESPONSES TO NEGATIVE SELF-TALK

TYPE OF SELF-TALK	SELF-DEFEATING THINKING	RIGHT THINKING
Externalizing/ Internalizing	My family is conspiring to keep me fat, so I can't lose weight.	Losing weight is within my control.
	I didn't lose weight this week; I must have screwed up.	I've reached an expected plateau. That's a good sign. My body is adjusting to the positive changes I've made.
Labeling	I'm a loser. I'm a failure.	Replace these thoughts with descriptions that are positive and accurately reflect who you are and what you stand for. Instead of a confining label, describe yourself positively, but always realistically. Call yourself a winner. Call yourself a runner. Call yourself a body-builder. Call yourself a health enthusiast—whatever, but describe yourself in a manner that reflects a winning identity.
Frustration Thinking	I'm so overwhelmed; I can't do it.	As long as I continue working on my weight, I'll achieve the goals I have set for myself.
Fortune-Telling	I will not succeed.	No matter what happens, I'll stay the course. If I do what is required, I will succeed.
All-or-Nothing Thinking	I've missed too many exercise classes. I'll just quit.	Quitting will get me nowhere. I'll analyze my schedule and make exercise a time-protected priority.

(continued on next page)

TYPE OF SELF-TALK	SELF-DEFEATING THINKING	RIGHT THINKING
Catastrophizing	I've gained two pounds, and it's terrible.	I'll review my week and see where I can improve. After all, since starting this program I've lost 20 pounds.
Pipe Dreaming	I'm going to lose five pounds this week.	I'll stick to my program, a day at a time. Whatever I lose will be a positive.
Gut-Level Reasoning	I feel fat, so I must look fat.	There's no evidence for this. I am looking better than ever.
Self-Downing	I hate my thighs.	I am learning to love my God-given body, and I love how I feel and look.
Poor Me Thinking	I can't have fun anymore.	Not true. The fitter I get, the more fun I have, and the more activities I can participate in. Life is more fun than ever.

To help you in this important work, please take out the Internal Audit assignment you completed at the very beginning of this chapter in which you recorded your thoughts about your appearance, your body shape, your ability to manage your weight, your exercise level, your self-control, and your general health. Review those messages, selecting the ones that are defeated and negative in tone. Transfer any that apply to the worksheet below.

Don't just breeze by this assignment, thinking about your answers in your mind. Instead, write them out so that you are coherent and consistent. Putting them down on paper, then analyzing them, will help you see whether they make sense or have any basis in fact.

To complete this assignment, use the chart on page 79. In the second column ("Self-Defeating Thinking"), record your self-talk as it pertains to the six subjects listed. Identify the type of self-talk you're expressing and list it in the first column ("Type of Self-Talk"). See pages 66 to 71 for help.

Then review your answers—the thoughts you recorded—for each of the six areas and test their validity. For each thought you recorded, ask:

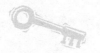

CHART 1. ANALYZE AND RESPOND TO YOUR SELF-TALK

1. Type of Self-Talk	2. Self-Defeating Thinking: What do you tell yourself about the following:	3. Validity	4. Right Thinking
	Your appearance:		
	Your body shape:		
	Your ability to manage your weight:		
	Your exercise level:		
	Your self-control:		
	Your general health:		

Is it true?

Is it in my best interest?

Does it protect my health?

Does it help me reach my goals?

Write your answers in the third column ("Validity") next to each instance of self-talk.

Finally, create positive balancing dialogue. For each self-defeating thought you recorded in column two, write an alternative thought that is positive, rational, and holds up to the truth of your weight-management efforts. Record this alternative thought in the fourth column ("Right Thinking"). Replacing negative internal dialogue with more constructive messages is an effective tool that can help you reduce the frequency and intensity of your negative self-talk.

As you go through this important exercise, tell yourself that you will probably add to this list over time, since you'll encounter challenges down the road, and will recognize on your internal radar other negative messages. Always be on the lookout, determined to unmask distortions and wrong thinking. Getting rid of negativism is a giant step toward achieving permanent weight loss and control.

You have completed some very vital work here. If wrong thinking has been infecting your life for a very long time, keep in mind that changing it is an ongoing process. You must seek to question your locus of control, dispute the inner conversations you have with yourself, come to grips with your self-honesty, and make it a matter of practice to replace self-abusive talk with rational, healthy dialogue. You must work hard to ensure that your thinking and your self-perceptions are not continually poisoned by faulty thinking. Be patient with yourself as you go through this process, because these are new skills that you are learning, and like any new skill, you master them only through practice.

5

Key Two:
Healing Feelings

Unlock the Door to
Emotional Control

We acquire the strength we have overcome.
—Ralph Waldo Emerson

Key #2: Healing feelings.

You make the choices that create your emotional state. Make them in a rational, purposeful way, and you will stop the cycle of emotional overeating that has for too long perpetuated your weight problem.

This key unlocks the door to emotional control so that you can quit looking to food for the answers to your emotional pain. They're not there. The solutions lie within you. This key gives you the power to heal your feelings so that your eating behavior is no longer fueled by harmful emotions.

Everyone—you are no exception—has an irrational and destructive emotional side to their personalities that rears its ugly head during times of trouble: unpaid bills, wayward kids, marriage turmoil, job stress, and more. You sink into depression or become unglued with stress, you lash out, you spew out venomous things you wish you hadn't, you are bitter and resentful, and you live with guilt and shame, and these emotions influence the way you behave. It is during those emotionally charged moments in life, that these feelings can trigger emotional overeating.

Almost instinctively, when we feel stress, anxiety, or depression, it is a natural human impulse to turn to food—and for a physiologically based reason. It is a long-established fact of nutritional science that food affects the brain's synthesis of certain natural chemicals, and that these chemicals have a stabilizing effect on mood and mental functioning. The problem is that in these moments we tend to reach for foods such as cookies, cake, candy, or ice cream—so-called "comfort foods"—all stuff that is so at odds with effective weight control. For many people, foods like these can be as fiendish as cigarettes, drugs, or alcohol, summoning up a loss of control that resembles the behavior of addiction, and they can be just as difficult to give up. Physiologically, these foods excite the same circuits in your brain that are stimulated by pleasure-inducing drugs, delivering a mild and short-lived high.

Habitually using food as a drug in order to cope with emotional pain and stress can quickly overtake you and become an addiction, with such terrible side effects as weight gain, poor body image, and severe self-esteem problems. When you routinely abuse food as an opiate, eating inappropriately, you leave yourself with a residue of guilt, depression, and more stress and anxiety. A vicious cycle ensues.

Never in your life will you be without emotional pain and stress—problems, challenges, and difficult moments are simply a part of living. You know that if things are going well at work, for example, you can count on conflict at home, or vice versa. There is rarely a time in your life when all is at peace and balance. That's neither good nor bad; it is simply the ebb and flow of how life works. To be alive means to experience emotions, painful or otherwise.

Living with unchecked emotional pain, however, sucks the pleasure out of life. It is absolutely incompatible with everything you want, need, and deserve, including proper weight management, good health, an active life, peace, and joy. This is why regaining emotional control in your life is one of the most important things you can do in order to stay the course without giving up on what you want. Once you start using this key, with its corresponding steps, you will start feeling good about who you are and what you want. You will begin to take control of your weight, as a result. There is more for you out there than reactive, destructive stress eating. I am going to show you how to get it. With this key, we will focus on how emotional overeating happens, how it gets to you, and what to do about it.

EMOTIONAL AUDITS

More than 50 percent of all overweight people use food to cope with depression, anger, stress, and other emotions. Are you among them? Are you? Because you can't change what you don't acknowledge, let's pause right here and begin to find out with our next audit, entitled "Are You an Emotional Eater?" As with the other self-tests you've taken so far, please be brutally honest in your answers. Let nothing emerge unexamined. You must find out the extent to which emotions are driving your eating behavior, because allowing emotionality to lord it over your behavior will cause you to fail—not some of the time, but all of the time.

ARE YOU AN EMOTIONAL EATER?

Look through the following questions. Check off the reasons you eat on various occasions, according to whether the statement is a frequent cause for you to eat, it serves as an occasional reason; or it never serves as a cause to eat. Answer all 25 questions.

REASON	FREQUENTLY	OCCASIONALLY	NEVER
1. I munch when I get bored.	( )	( )	( )
2. I like to eat with my friends, even if I am not hungry.	( )	( )	( )
3. I eat so the cook will not be offended.	( )	( )	( )
4. I eat when I get depressed.	( )	( )	( )
5. I eat when I am lonely.	( )	( )	( )

(continued on next page)

REASON	FREQUENTLY	OCCASIONALLY	NEVER
6. I eat when I get anxious about something.	( )	( )	( )
7. There are times when my eating is out of control.	( )	( )	( )
8. I like to nurture other people with food.	( )	( )	( )
9. I will eat my way through a difficult time (divorce, job loss, illness, broken dream).	( )	( )	( )
10. I eat when I feel my energy go down.	( )	( )	( )
11. I crave some foods.	( )	( )	( )
12. I just like to have something in my mouth.	( )	( )	( )
13. I eat even if I am not hungry.	( )	( )	( )
14. I like to celebrate with food.	( )	( )	( )
15. I think about food a good deal of the time.	( )	( )	( )
16. I have a tendency to binge.	( )	( )	( )
17. I eat to be polite.	( )	( )	( )
18. I am embarrassed sometimes by how much I eat.	( )	( )	( )
19. I eat to relax myself and relieve stress.	( )	( )	( )

REASON	FREQUENTLY	OCCASIONALLY	NEVER
20. I get upset if I overeat.	( )	( )	( )
21. I eat because I get angry.	( )	( )	( )
22. I am displeased with my weight, but I overeat anyway.	( )	( )	( )
23. I eat everything that is placed in front of me and always clean my plate, so as not to waste food.	( )	( )	( )
24. I need high levels of sugar in my system.	( )	( )	( )
25. Eating is my main enjoyment in life.	( )	( )	( )

SCORING

For each "frequently" you checked, give yourself 2 points; for each "occasionally," give yourself 1 point; and for each "never," give yourself 0 points. Total your points for a score in the range of 0 to 50. This is your "emotional eating" score.

Interpretation

This audit is designed to give you a quick snapshot of whether or not you are an emotional eater. If your overall score (your emotional eating score) is more than 35, it is likely that you have serious trouble with emotional eating, and regardless of what else is working, you must get the self-defeating nature of your emotions under control. If your score is between 15 and 35, you struggle with emotional eating at times, and you have room for improvement. There may be isolated areas, such as stress or depression, in which you can change.

STRESS AUDIT

Stress-induced overeating is certainly a major cause of weight gain—and not only because of the excess calories you consume when medicating yourself with food. Stress—particularly when it is prolonged and unresolved—provokes weight-sustaining physiological changes in your body. When you are under stress, your body releases hormones that automatically stimulate your appetite and set off cravings, prompting you to eat huge quantities of fattening food.

Understand this too: stress attacks your health in other ways, particularly if you allow it to stack up. Heaps of unresolved stress have far worse consequences than weight gain. Stress can take years off your life and make you more susceptible to disease. How? If you are constantly under stress, your body's natural immune defenses are dramatically disrupted because of the close communication between your immune cells and your nerve cells, and a defeating physiology occurs. It might take the form of tension headaches, migraines, fatigue, backaches, sleep disturbances, ulcers, elevated blood pressure, even heart attacks.

Thus, the next audit I want you to take is an inventory of stressors in your life—those events or situations that have the potential to rob you of health, peace, and joy if you let them. Stressors are what they are: they're a part of life; they happen. They come and go; they scram or stay. It's important to identify and consciously acknowledge your stressors so that you can begin to work on reducing them to manageable levels. Let's get started on this next important audit.

STRESS SCALE

Check off the stressors that you have experienced in the last twelve months:

1. (95) Death of a child

2. (93) Divorce

3. (90) Death of a spouse

4. (80) Death of a parent

5. (80)   Spouse's or partner's betrayal of trust

6. (80)   New marriage

7. (75)   Job change after age of 45

8. (70)   Conflict between you and your spouse

9. (70)   Conflict with boss where job is threatened

10. (65)   Significant negative medical diagnosis

11. (55)   Change of home location

12. (50)   Retirement

13. (50)   Conflict between you and your teenager

14. (50)   Conflict between you and a parent

15. (40)   40th, 50th, 60th, 75th, or 80th birthdays

16. (35)   Significant traumatic injury (include heart attack if appropriate)

17. (35)   Having to commit parent to assisted-care home or facility

18. (30)   Job change

19. (30)   Marriage of daughter

20. (25)   Chronic pain condition

21. (25)   Best friend's betrayal of trust

22. (25)   Last child leaving home

23. (20)   Purchase of a new car or house

24. (20)   Big family celebration or get-together

25. (10)   Overly-demanding job responsibilities

SCORING AND INTERPRETATION

The number in the parentheses indicates the average intensity of stress on a scale from 10 (low stress) to 95 (paralyzing stress). For the stressors you checked, add up the corresponding numbers.

If your score is between 0 and 30, you are under very little stress at present and very likely have good physical and mental health.

If your score ranges from 35 to 65, the stress in your life may begin to undermine your weight loss efforts and harm your overall health.

A score above 65 indicates that you are undergoing significant stress, and this may initiate bouts of overeating as well as disease-causing changes in your biochemistry. You need support and must work toward acquiring some very specific tools of stress management.

REGAINING EMOTIONAL CONTROL

There you are: slumped in your easy chair, scarfing down a box of Twinkies, feeling sorry for yourself because your marriage is boring, your kids are demanding, or your job is stressful. And however much you wish you didn't cope like this, you continue to do it, time after time.

One of the most critical ways to stop this behavior is to change the way you think and how you interpret events in your life. What you think determines how you feel. So if you want to change your feelings about something—and the negative behavior that flows from those feelings—then you must change and reshape the thought patterns that are making you sad, anxious, lonely, or depressed.

Many of our thought patterns are shaped through individual "filters." These filters—our personalities, attitudes, points of view, and beliefs—are internal screening devices that affect how we see the world and react to it. Largely a product of our past experiences, our filters powerfully influence the interpretation we give to the events in our lives. Those interpretations, in turn, determine how we will respond to life. To illustrate this concept for you in a simple, understandable way, refer to the familiar biblical story of David and Goliath. When the Israelite soldiers first set eyes on Goliath, their reaction was: "He is so big that we can never slay him." When David saw Goliath, he said to himself, "He is so big that I cannot miss him." Two completely different reactions to the very same stressor, because of very different perceptual filters.

You probably know people like those soldiers who, when confronted with emotionally charged situations or stress, are prone to panic, disconnect, or fall to pieces. Life just seems to drive them around the bend. By contrast, you probably know other people, like David in the example, who actually seem to thrive on stress and do their best work under pressure. I can't emphasize this enough: two poles apart reactions can occur in response to the very same set of stimuli. Why? Because one person runs the stress through a filter that causes it to be perceived as overwhelming and impossible to handle, while the other person's filter says, "This is a problem I can turn into an opportunity."

When you consider the relevance of this observation to your own emotional management, you begin to see that your interpretation of the event, not so much the event itself, is the real trouble-maker that gets you so worked up. You will always be challenged by stressors in your life. The tire is flat. Your boss is a jerk. Money may be tight. Your boyfriend didn't call when he said he would. The diagnosis wasn't good. The person you married fifteen years ago took off. Yes, these things are bad, but it is your interpretation of and reaction to them that create the emotional pain. Worse yet, avoiding these emotions instead of dealing constructively with them will tax your body and your health, so much so that you may shorten your life by years and years.

There is another type of filter that creates more trouble and stress than you can imagine. This filter is the filter of denial. You might, for example, think that your weight problem is just cosmetic. Yes, being heavy affects your appearance, but you would never admit that it puts you at risk for premature death from heart disease, stroke, cancer, or other life-shortening diseases, even though you're huffing and puffing with every step. You're in severe denial that there are health problems connected with obesity. Or maybe you're vomiting up food to manage your out-of-control eating. You tell yourself you don't really have an eating disorder; you're just engaging in this behavior temporarily, until you achieve your ideal weight or solve the stress in your life. You're denying that you are suffering from an eating disorder, and you avoid facing up to the problem.

Denial is a dangerous filter because it suppresses the truth about yourself. Living in denial, you can be like a pressure cooker that is not allowed to vent its steam. All this pressure builds up inside you—

until the lid blows off or the pot cracks at its weakest point. Denying certain realities weakens us, and kills what might have been a real chance to overcome a problem, had the solution been pursued in time. If you continue to view your eating problems through a filter of denial, then you are allowing self-deception to control and dictate your behavior, then days, weeks, months, and years will continue to be wasted: time that could and would have been amazing and significant in your life.

As information flows through your filters, it takes the form of words. It becomes a dialogue, a conversation you have with yourself. As we saw in the previous chapter, a lot of this mental activity happens in real time; this is your self-talk. It often contains errors in thinking that can lead to emotional problems unless these errors are dragged out into the open, disputed, and restructured.

Another type of faulty mental activity—termed *automatic thoughts*—goes on in your mind, too. Automatic thoughts happen so fast, so repetitively, that we are often unaware of them. They are activated automatically in response to your interpretation of a particular event or situation. Remember, your interpretation—the meaning you assign to a situation—is what triggers your emotional response, as opposed to the event that has actually taken place. Your emotions flow from the meaning you attach to situations.

If you have repeatedly assigned the same meaning to certain events, then your thoughts, your interpretations of those events, are predictably going to be the same every time. Those thoughts will eventually become habitual and automatic, to the point that you're no longer aware of them. You've programmed and conditioned yourself to think and behave the same way whenever certain situations arise.

For example, suppose someone in your family criticizes you. Without your really being aware of them, automatic thoughts like "They never approve of me" or "they just won't accept me as I am" start racing through your mind. In response, you feel hurt, and before you know it, you're spooning ice cream into your mouth right out of the carton. You probably didn't know what you were thinking when you got criticized, but the next thing you knew, you were bingeing on ice cream. Why? Feeling hurt was preceded by negative, lightning-speed thoughts you have always had, thoughts you internalized long ago, whenever you were criticized by your family. These thoughts are so overlearned, and happening so fast, that you are not consciously aware of how they affect your behavior. Your behavior is being controlled by an internal negative attitude that you can't even recognize.

The question arises: if that's the case, what can I do about it? The good news is that these thoughts, like your real-time self-talk, can be controlled, challenged, and changed. By changing the way you think, you can change the way you feel and act. What you're about to do, in the following series of steps, will help you change your emotional state so that you no longer medicate yourself with food in emotionally charged situations.

STEP ONE: TAKE OWNERSHIP OF YOUR REACTIONS

Review the stress audit you just took, looking over the stressors that are listed. In truth, no event, no person, not one of the situations listed on the stress scale can "stress you out" and make you eat a box of doughnuts; what initiates stress and anxiety is your response to the stressor. Remember, you respond not to what happens in the world (external events), but instead to your interpretation of those events. In other words, it is what you think about and how you evaluate an event that determines how you feel, as well as what you do in response.

Suppose, for example, that you apply for a job that you really wanted, but you are not hired. That is an external event to which you had some internal reaction. It is your internal reaction to not being hired that impacts your emotions, not the actual event. Let's say your internal reaction is, "Hey, I don't like getting turned down. But I know in my heart I am a talented, capable, and competent employee, and I will apply for another job." You are being rational, realistic, and you are not likely to get upset and suffer a huge blow to your self-worth.

On the other hand, maybe your internal reaction is, "I'm such a loser. I blew the interview, it was so humiliating, and I got what I deserved. That job was too good for me, and I'm really not good enough to even apply for it. They knew I couldn't cut it. Give me a bag of chips so I can feel better."

What happens in the wake of that thinking is a feeling of stress, or maybe some other emotion like depression. You believe that not getting the job made you upset, when in fact, it was your thinking about the situation that hurt you. Not getting the job isn't what upset you; it is the thoughts you have about the situation that are causing the emotional pain.

Whatever the situation, you can choose your reaction. No matter what the circumstances, your interpretation of those events is of your own choosing. The events in your daily life have only the meaning you assign to them. This is why one of my life laws states "There is no reality, only perception." How you interpret the events, circumstances, and situations in your life is entirely up to you.

If your response is counterproductive, test your perceptions more often and become more accountable for how you react to the stress and problems in your life. Stop being overly sensitive to the negatives while filtering out the positives. Maintain an active, ongoing awareness of your reactions, and recognize where your outlook is distorted so that you can make adjustments.

Make no mistake: I am not suggesting that one of your choices is to interpret everything that happens to you in a Pollyanna fashion. Obviously, that would not always be a rational reaction. Should you experience one of life's top stressors—the death of a child, or a divorce—it is not rational for you to interpret that in any way as being good. However, you do have a choice about whether that event will be your absolute undoing, or whether it becomes something you deal with in a constructive manner. The latter choice means that you will create meaning and purpose out of your suffering; that can take any number of forms, from becoming a counselor to other victims of a similar tragedy to volunteering for a cause. The most important choice you have in light of a personal tragedy is what you do now. The past is over. The future hasn't happened yet. The only time is now.

STEP TWO: RESOLVE, RATHER THAN REACT TO, LIFE'S PROBLEMS

Take a problem-solving approach to emotion-provoking events. Commit to resolving rather than enduring the problems that contribute to your stress, anxiety, or depression. You can either sit around and stew about the situation, or you can make the choice to be self-directed, take action, and adopt a solution-side approach to your life. If it's a bill you can't pay, whining and worrying about it won't satisfy your creditor. If it's a sales call you blew, beating yourself up over it won't help you meet your quota. If it's an argument with your spouse, withdrawing, pouting, and barricading yourself behind a locked bedroom door won't bring things to resolution. What's more, none of these situations will get better if you respond by stuffing yourself with uncontrolled amounts of food. Food is not a fix-it-all.

Ask yourself: do I just react to what's in my face, or do I act? Stop living reactively and begin to choose the right attitude and the right behavior to generate the right results. Remember that it is action—not reaction—that gets meaningful, constructive results. So take charge because problems almost never resolve themselves; they don't get better with inattention. Once you start acting instead of reacting, you'll realize that those old sayings have long lives because they are true: "No one ever climbed a hill just by looking at it." "You can't get anywhere unless you start." "All things come to him who goes after it." When you are accountable for your problems and for their solutions, you are an agent of change.

STEP THREE: DECELERATE YOUR THINKING

Changing your emotional response, and the unwanted eating behavior that flows from it, requires slowing down, listening carefully to your thinking, evaluating your reactions, and altering those reactions.

That is why you must learn to decelerate your thinking—put your mind into slow motion like a videotape or film—so that you can cause everything to go at a steady, deliberate pace. I know this sounds like a tall order, but let me assure you that it will be one of the easiest and most effective ways to manage your emotional life.

If you have open emotional wounds, if your "psychological skin" has been burned, then you *will* "feed the need." Food can be a great comforter, a great distracter, and create weight that is a great excuse to drop out of all or part of your life.

Sandra, a former patient of mine, was a tragic but clear example. At 5 feet, 2 inches and 195 pounds, she professed to be desperate to lose weight. Yet, despite repeated attempts at dieting, all with partial success, she would invariably "crater" every single time she got close to her goal. Consciously, Sandra hated her appearance and actually feared for her life, knowing that she was a high risk for heart attack and stroke. Sandra could recite to me everything there was to know about losing weight, eating right, and exercising. But, seemingly without rhyme or reason, Sandra would actually sabotage herself. She wanted the results—until she got close, and then she seemed to choke.

It was clear to me that Sandra was getting some kind of payoff, or reward, for this self-sabotage. Somehow, some way, she unconsciously felt unworthy or uncomfortable with giving up her obesity and claiming victory. I began to dig and dig deep, and it didn't take long to solve the mystery.

Starting at age ten, Sandra had begun to go through puberty and show the outward signs of becoming a young woman—changes that did not go unnoticed by a sick and depraved uncle who sexually molested her. The violation continued for years, and these were years marked by the shame and guilt of a naïve and confused little girl. Blaming herself and her body for the unwanted attention and feelings that her changing figure had seemingly attracted, Sandra soon became uncomfortable and ashamed of her sexuality. She soon discovered that, as she inadvertently put on weight, the attention seemed to lessen. As she became more obese, her secondary sexual characteristics were in a sense camouflaged, and a feeling of safety came upon her.

Sandra and I began to see that remaining overweight insulated her from the attentions of the opposite sex. Every time she would approach her goal and begin to receive compliments from men, panic ensued, and she retreated to the safety of her camouflage. Sandra's self-sabotage was, in fact, a return to shelter by putting back on the weight she had lost. Her payoff for remaining obese was safety from men and from the feelings of anxiety that their attention fostered. Although that "shelter" offered a temporary haven, Sandra's panic would eventually diminish, the pain of obesity would burn hottest again, and she would start another diet and lose weight, only to relapse whenever asked out for a date or complimented. This vicious circle continued relentlessly, with no hope of stopping because the need for the weight had never been eliminated.

I asked Sandra to slow her thoughts down, relax, and recall the painful incidents with her uncle, and to tell me what messages were going on in her head. With practice and repeated sessions, she started listening to what had become well-rehearsed, internal, automatic activity. I asked her to write down these statements, and we reviewed them. She was shocked by what she had been telling herself: "I'm dirty. I'm disgusting. I'm damaged goods. I'm just another piece of garbage on the heap that no man would want for other than sex. I'm afraid and ashamed of intimacy. *I need my weight as a place to hide.*" With jolting clarity, Sandra realized that her "unhealed" feelings held her prisoner. She *needed* that weight and as long as she did, neither a diet nor a program would ever be allowed to take it away from her. How about you? Do you *need* your weight as a coping mechanism? Are you self-sabotaging for some unapparent reason?

You must go through the same process in which I guided Sandra. Slow your thoughts down, and listen attentively. That way, you'll be able to hear what you are thinking. You do this by becoming very still and very quiet, and recording your thoughts. These high-speed thoughts and internal reactions always precede your feelings and emotions. Trust me, you did tell yourself something if you now feel angry, mad, anxious, frustrated, sad, or depressed. From now on, whenever you get upset, listen ever so carefully to what you are telling yourself.

Be sure to write your thoughts down. If all you do is just think them through, there will be no impact. Writing them helps you appraise your thoughts more objectively and allows you to get some distance from them. Think of what you record as a mirror. Just as it would be impossible to study your own face without a mirror, it is impossible to study your own life without writing it down. So: write it down!

STEP FOUR: CHALLENGE AND RESTRUCTURE YOUR AUTOMATIC THOUGHTS

Once you identify what is going on in your mind, work to change it. If you now get it that emotional pain stems from your thoughts, then you must correct the errors in your thinking. By overriding your mental conditioning, you can reprogram yourself and better manage your emotional life. With the first key—right thinking—you began this critically important process by asking yourself four questions regarding your internal dialogue, and you must do the same in disputing your automatic thoughts:

Are they true?

Do they serve your best interests?

Do they advance and protect your health?

Do they help you achieve your weight-management goals?

Once again, answer these hard questions about how you think and what you believe about yourself. When you start to test them against reality, your beliefs and attitudes will begin to change in rather short measure, no matter how long-standing they are. By using this line of questioning on your thoughts and beliefs—testing them against reality—you can change your perceptions, your judgments, and your evaluations of yourself. Until you stop and analyze your internal reactions, you will go on believing them and continuing to deal with these emotions that are so much at war with your best self. So the paramount issue for you is that you have to understand how you work, from the inside out, and what makes you feel the way you feel.

To be liberated from the control of negative emotions, you'll need to continue to do a fair amount of the introspection I've been describing here. You have to see the truth in the fact that you are responsible for upsetting yourself. It is wrong to continue in the belief that something or someone is causing you to feel emotions you do not want to feel. I know I keep knocking this into your head: you can't change other people or other conditions; you can change only your reactions to them.

That's why you'll have to identify the irrational thoughts and beliefs that you continually and automatically send yourself. And you will have to sort through these messages, restructure them, and replace them with authentic responses that correct your high-speed thinking, just as you did with faulty internal dialogue in the last chapter. Only by counterattacking your self-criticisms can you better control the emotions that are keeping your unwanted eating behavior alive.

In Sandra's case, she had to restructure her thinking by healing her feelings of pain, fear, and anxiety that came from sexual relevancy. Sandra had to say, "I now know that I was used and abused, and that it was not my fault. Nor was it the fault of being an attractive and healthy woman. It is not bad, disgusting, or dirty to be thin, vibrant, and alive. I have to stop judging myself. I did nothing wrong.

I am worthy of dignity, respect, and love. I am here for myself, and I accept the qualities that make me beautiful and special." When she was able to adopt a new view of herself, the destructive emotional responses that formerly flowed from her thinking began to fade. She broke the vicious cycle.

You must get in touch with your thoughts and feelings and why you're having them. If you're unwilling to investigate your true feelings in order to give them a voice, then you will continue to stumble along in life, with an absolute guarantee of failure and frustration. Have the courage to ask yourself the hard questions, and to give the answers an appropriate voice. Get real with yourself. Be willing to be introspective enough to identify and admit what is really going on with you.

When conflict arises, or when you're walking through an emotional minefield, as you know you will, don't panic and seek solace in food. Have an emotional plan in place for how you will deal with and respond to the situation. You will simply say to yourself, "I will control what attitude I take toward this situation. I have the power to choose my perceptions and my reactions. And I will exercise this power of choice in every circumstance, every day of my life."

STEP FIVE: GAIN EMOTIONAL CLOSURE

If you allow ugly emotions to take root in your heart and mind, they will not remain specific to the situation that provoked them. They begin to contaminate all your relationships and all your interactions with other people. Who you once were dies away, and now you are defined by these ugly emotions. What ultimately makes these emotions so powerful is that they change who you are. They change what you do and contaminate what you give.

With this powerful truth in mind, I think you can see why you must refuse to live with unfinished emotional business. As long as you do, it will consume you. Maintaining anger, hurt, vengeance, hatred, and other negative emotional burdens eats away at your body, as it does your soul. It is just so easy, in a busy and ever-changing life, to allow emotional pain and discord to accumulate. But heaps of unfinished emotional business can crush your self-control, and you will self-medicate, again and again, with ever-increasing amounts of food.

If emotional pain or problems have cropped up in your life, you must insist on getting closure. Closure means you don't carry the problem or the pain. You address the issue, then you slam shut the book and put it away. Whatever that takes, do it. Whatever it requires, you do it to get past it. You must avoid piling up this kind of burden in your life; you must give yourself emotional closure.

The emotions I'm describing here are the open wounds of unfinished emotional business with somebody, somewhere: a person or persons who is the target of all that negative emotion. If you bear the unhealed scars of hatred, anger, resentment, and bitterness, you are doing so because you have never gotten emotional closure on the treatment you got at the hands of that other person. You and only you choose how you feel. Others may provide an event or behavior for you to react to, but it is up to you to choose how you feel about them. If you choose to carry the hatred, then know that you choose to experience the world in a dark way, and you're all the more likely to medicate yourself with food.

The goal of this step is to help you gain important emotional closure so that you can resolve your situation and its associated pain, and prevent potential relapses into behavior that keeps you from attaining your weight-management goals. A powerful process that I use to help people get emotional closure is what I call your Minimal Effective Response (MER). The operative word here is "minimal," meaning the least thing you can do to get emotional closure.

So that you fully understand this concept, let me explain what MER is not. For one thing, it is not seeking revenge, or plotting ways to undermine other people. Taking such actions only harms you in the long run because you are still holding on to self-destructive emotions. A rattlesnake, if cornered, can become so enraged that it will bite itself. That is no different from what we do when we choose to harbor hate, vengeance, and grudges toward other people: we bite ourselves.

MER seeks to satisfy your need for emotional resolution without creating a whole new set of problems. Maybe it means confronting yourself or the other person. Maybe it means taking legal action. Maybe it requires forgiveness or making an apology. Maybe it means writing a letter to someone, or stomping on a wrongdoer's grave. Maybe it involves seeing a mental health counselor, talking to your pastor or minister, or turning the situation and its emotional battle over to God. There are many different ways to obtain MER; the key is to get maximum results for minimal expense. When you initiate your MER, trust me, it will lessen your need to use food as medication.

To map out how you will execute your MER, you can use the following questions:

- What action can you take to resolve your emotional pain?

- If you are successful and achieve this resolution, how will you feel?

- Does the feeling you will have match the feeling you want to have?

- Remembering the word "minimal," could there be some other economical action that would give you the emotional resolution you need?

Turning again to Sandra, she would consider possible MERs by asking herself: what is the least thing I could do to get justice, to heal the emotional wounds I suffered at the hands of my uncle? Maybe she needs to go to him, look him in the eye, and tell him, "Don't you think for one minute that I don't know what you did to me, it is illegal, and I want to be heard. You need to know how that hurt me. You need to know how it has affected my life."

Maybe that's her MER. Maybe she needs the cathartic effect of having that confrontation. On the other hand, maybe that won't do it for her. Maybe Sandra needs to take advantage of the fact that there is no statute of limitations on molestation and go to the authorities. Maybe that is what she needs to do.

After considering your own emotional responses, and the nature and degree of the suffering you have endured, what is your MER? Maybe you don't have the energy or resources to take legal action. Maybe all you need to do is compose a letter and write down all your thoughts and feelings. Maybe that MER will work for you. Maybe you need to mail the letter, if your situation involves another person. But whatever your MER is, you need to identify it and you need to do it.

You need to say, "Okay, it's done. I've had enough. I will no longer allow you to rob me of my self-control. I'm shutting the book on this. My emotional business is finished, and I am free to go back to being that person that I now know I am."

THE POWER OF FORGIVENESS

There is one more facet to this vitally important action called MER: the key with which you unlock your emotional prison and set yourself free may be a minimally effective response called forgiveness. Initially, forgiveness may be very hard for you, because you feel that it demonstrates weakness rather than strength. I submit to you that this powerful human act does anything but, and it may be absolutely essential in order for you to gain emotional closure and make positive change.

Let's be clear about what I mean when I use the word *forgiveness*: I'm talking about something that happens entirely within you. Forgiveness is a choice, a choice that you make to release yourself from the emotional prison of anger, hatred, and resentment. I am not saying that the choice is an easy one, only that it is a necessary one. You should also know that when I use the word forgiveness, I in no way mean that I am asking you to take the position that whatever may have happened to you in your life is now okay. Forgiveness is not a feeling that you passively wait to come over you. It is a choice you make.

Another one of my life laws states, "There is power in forgiveness." The reason is that, without forgiveness, you are destined to lug around your emotional burdens, and suffer emotional and physical consequences as a result. You may believe right now that you are justified to hate, or harbor rage, against someone who has hurt you deeply enough to create these emotions. You may believe that they deserve it and should be made to suffer by your hatred of them. But to carry around these beliefs is to pay an unbelievably high price, because those feelings can become so pervasive as to contaminate every element of your current life.

When Leonardo da Vinci was working on his masterpiece *The Last Supper*, he became angry with a certain man. As his temper flared, he spewed out bitter words to the poor man. Afterwards, da Vinci returned to his painting and tried to work on the face of Jesus, but was so consumed by his anger that he could not compose himself for the meticulous work that was required. Finally, he laid aside his painting tools, sought out the man, and asked for forgiveness. The man accepted his apology and da Vinci was able to finish painting the face of Jesus.

Do you see the damage that an unforgiving spirit can inflict? Anger, hatred, and resentment become all-consuming, so much so that they become a part of your every waking hour. By not forgiving your wrongdoers, you allow them to lock you back into your prison, and they win. You see: forgiveness of those who have transgressed against you, or those you love, is not about them; it is about you.

If you are unsure as to how to forgive—if you are unsure about what to say within your heart—let me help you give a voice to your choice of forgiveness. You might say the following to yourself:

I am making a choice to forgive you. By doing so, I free myself from the bond I had with you through hatred, anger, resentment, or fear. I take my power back and gain the freedom that only forgiveness can bring. You cannot hurt me and you cannot control me. I forgive for myself.

Trust me on this: the only escape from your particular emotional prison may truly be forgiveness. By making that choice, you rise above the pain to take the moral high ground and forgive the person who hurt you. Everything they have done to you, they have already done to themselves. If you allow people who have wronged you to keep you imprisoned, then they win. Don't worry about when or how they will "get theirs." Their judgment will not come from you, but ultimately from God, who settles all accounts.

Rethink the meaning of forgiveness, and set yourself free from the emotional pain that has been inflicted on you by others in your life. This may be one of the most important things you learn in this chapter. Don't wait another day. You have the ability to forgive those people—not as a gift to them, but as a gift to yourself. Forgive them, start healing, and get on with your life.

COPING WITHOUT FOOD

Before leaving this key, let me talk to you about a coping tool that, if built into the day-to-day flow of your life, will begin to restore peace and tranquillity, and keep you from turning to food for solace from emotional pain. If you're upset and treat yourself to a plate of cookies or a bag of candy because you "deserve it," get real. There are other ways to treat yourself and restore calm without resorting to a food binge. That's why you must carve out time in your life for tension-reducing activities. I suspect that if you habitually overeat in reaction to stress or emotional pain, then you have no clue as to how to relax without a food binge. You are more accustomed to putting something fattening in your mouth to get relief than using nonfood activities to calm yourself down.

When your nerve cells become agitated by anxiety or depression, and by your mental response to this emotional state, it is not easy to quiet them down. Sure, you can do it quickly by resorting to chemical means such as tranquilizers or alcohol, or high-calorie comfort foods, but those are devastatingly counterproductive and will cause you to close the door to other positive alternatives that can be incredibly powerful.

These alternatives include, but are not limited to, working out (a powerful stress reliever!), performing relaxation exercises, and listening to music. By most research accounts, these activities work directly on your nervous system by releasing endorphins, your brain's natural tranquilizers, to produce a state of reduced anxiety and a feeling of calm. These activities are natural, nonchemical, and inexpensive relaxants.

When you consider various tension-reducing activities, I realize that you may not be open to relaxation exercises such deep breathing, yoga, or meditation. Maybe you think they won't help, or that they won't work. But what if something like this is exactly what you need when anxiety, stress, or depression strikes? What if it is?

When you are tense and under stress, there are corresponding and instantaneous responses in your physical body. One is a tightening of your stomach muscles and your diaphragm, a large sheet of muscle located at the bottom of your chest cavity, that is used for breathing. You begin to breathe in a shallow manner, and this creates even more tension. But by deep breathing, which is a type of relaxation exercise, you can release this tension and become more mentally focused on resolving the stress.

Now don't lock up on me here. This isn't Eastern mystical stuff. It's a quick, practical way to relax, and you can do it anywhere—at your desk, in an airplane, in your car, before you give a speech, or make an important sales call, wherever—and you can do it without anyone knowing. All it involves is taking fuller and deeper breaths, inhaling and exhaling through your nose very slowly and letting your chest rise and fall in a steady rhythm. In less than a minute, your diaphragm loosens. Your brain senses this, interprets it, and begins to release endorphins that further reduce the tension level in your body. Pretty soon, your tension is gone; you've pushed out all that is possible, and you're in the realm of relaxation. (In Appendix A, you will find instructions and a script for how to go about achieving stress reduction in this manner.)

Now you may be thinking, "Relaxation, breathing exercises, are you kidding? Give me something to eat!"

Please understand: now is not the time to be judgmental, resisting some tools that may genuinely help you. If you pooh-pooh this now, you may be cheating yourself later.

To help you see the power in these techniques, let me introduce to you my sister-in-law Cindi, who, as a single mom, raised three successful daughters and worked three jobs to send them all through college. She gave me permission to include her story, and I offer it as an example of how being open-minded to new and different techniques of coping can be life-changing in their effect. I am willing to bet that in a heartbeat her story may erase any doubt or mistrust you have over the techniques I am recommending here.

CINDI'S STORY

It began one morning in June of 2001. Just before sunrise, Cindi was being driven by her friend Jim to the airport in Oklahoma City, two hours away from her small-town home. She had won a trip from her employer based on her excellent performance in cable advertising sales, and was now on her way to enjoy the vacation. As they traveled, the country roads were empty; the morning was still.

Then the horror struck.

From an overpass, some madman or madmen dumped a vat of acid on the passenger side of the car. It crashed through the windshield, dousing Cindi on virtually every side with a torturous liquid fire. After swiftly disintegrating her clothing, the acid next ate at her flesh, melting and peeling away her skin, to burn more than 70 percent of her body, including her face, eyes, scalp, mouth, her entire torso, and the front of her legs.

Miles from anywhere and without water, Jim drove at lightning speed to find help, while the acid continued its relentless assault on Cindi's flesh and left her screaming in agony. Jim pulled in to an open gas station and called 911. Heroically, he began splashing water over Cindi, trying desperately to wash the burning acid from her face, eyes, and body, during those interminable minutes awaiting the arrival of an ambulance.

Nothing could have prepared Cindi for what she was now to face in the months that followed this act of cruel, senseless violence.

So began more than a dozen brutal reconstructive surgeries, including skin graphs, and the replacement of her eyelids, chin, and upper chin. Twice a day, her burns had to be cleansed so that infection would not grow, and her body could heal itself. It was a trial no human should have to go through.

The physical pain was slow, excruciating torment, unbearable, debilitating, and hellish. More unspeakable was the destruction of her life, the end of her world as she knew it.

At first, some modicum of relief came in the form of painkillers, but these could exact their own hell. Fearing addiction to painkillers, Cindi turned to me for help. I enlisted the aid of my mentor, G. Frank Lawlis, Ph.D., who is one of the leading authorities in the nation today in body-mind control. He designed a three-part program for Cindi that involved special relaxation and deep breathing exercises to help her overcome her fears and begin the healing process; calming techniques that helped her control her pain and deal with the emotional scars of the tragedy; and visual imagery, so that she could see her skin accepting the grafts and becoming as new as an infant's. Cindi had little confidence in these methods, initially. But her attitude changed—and changed dramatically.

Cindi recently told me that had it not been for Dr. Lawlis's help she never would have made it, that she would have given up living. Further, the program he designed for her dramatically accelerated her healing—to the utter amazement of her physicians. Cindi confessed that her own judgmental nature had almost cheated her out of this absolutely life-saving intervention.

For a very dear and beloved woman, this trip of terror turned into a life of triumph. Had she chosen to let the person or persons who committed this horrible act continue to haunt her, she would have engulfed herself in bitterness, only to empower the perpetrators to hurt her a second time around. But she did not. Every day that she awakens, Cindi feels blessed for the incredible day she has with her daughters and grandchildren, and thankful to God for every new day of living.

There is certainly much more to her story, especially about how Cindi came back to life physically, emotionally, and spiritually, but I will leave it at that.

My message to you right now is simply this: guard against being closed-minded; do not slam your ears shut. Your challenge is to consider all the possible coping skills available to you other than eating, that will bring you the payoffs of peace and balance in your life.

So if you want to succeed in losing weight, get out of your comfort zone and be open to trying new ways to manage stress, anxiety, and other painful emotions. Be willing to plunge into the unknown, if necessary, leaving behind the safe, unchallenging, and familiar existence, in order to have more. Take a new direction and change your life.

As you incorporate more tension-reducing activities in your life, please continue to work hard on your underlying reactions and responses to stress and emotional pain, and change them so that you become less reactive. This will help you manage your emotions in the long run; there is no doubt about it. Even so, something as simple as breathing deeply will help you calm down so that you can at least examine and evaluate your reaction to the pain or stress, so that your thinking can stay focused and you will avoid medicating yourself with food.

Learning to better manage your emotions often greatly reduces not only the frequency and intensity of those emotions, but also the number of times you slide back into the old self-destructive patterns of overeating, bingeing, and other actions that run counter to weight management. You'll be astounded by how much more orderly, peaceful, and fulfilling your life will become. You'll push your emotional life to the best levels of who you are in your mind and heart. You'll have a newfound sense of freedom. You'll feel good about yourself and your body. You'll feel good about life, and you will live it to the fullest and best of your ability.

6

Key Three: A No-Fail Environment

Unlock the Door to External Control

Sometimes it is not good enough to do your best;
you have to do what's required.
—SIR WINSTON CHURCHILL

KEY #3: A NO-FAIL ENVIRONMENT.

You can't eat what's not there. When you reduce your exposure to food, you program yourself against out-of-control eating and make it practically impossible to fail at weight loss.

This key unlocks the door to *external control*. External control means that your environment—places like your home or office, anywhere you see food, think about food, store food, prepare food, sneak food, and eat food—is safe from problematic foods and reminders to eat. With external control, food is out of sight, out of reach, and out of mind.

Because many of you overeat because food is available and accessible, the best way to counter inappropriate, problematic eating is to change your exposure and access to food by rearranging and managing your external environment. A case in point: recently, I received letters from two women who took to heart my message that "You can't eat unhealthy food if it's not there." They decided to clean out their cupboards and refrigerators, and avoid fast-food restaurants and other places that did not support their weight loss goals. With these very simple changes in their lifestyle, these women lost 10 and 14 pounds, respectively, in only three weeks. As they did, you will find that weight loss becomes so much easier when you control your environment by eliminating opportunities that invite needless snacking, overeating, and bingeing.

This key has nothing to do with increasing willpower or trying to mentally resist food temptations, but rather with reengineering your environment in such a way that it "pulls for" the result that you desire. Any self-destructive behavior involving a "substance of choice," whether it is nicotine, alcohol, food, or something else, will manifest itself depending on the level of access to that substance in the environment. Remove access and you stand a better chance of quitting. As proof, there are documented cases of soldiers who became addicted to heroin in Vietnam, but upon returning home to a different environment, were able to permanently kick their habit.

That's why, in the same way, I can cure smoking, alcoholism, or drug addiction; I can cause addicts to defeat their addiction 100 percent of the time, provided I put them in an environment where there is no tobacco, alcohol, or drugs. Addiction cured. Realistically though, nothing short of parachuting them into the Antarctic will ensure such a temptation-free environment. But each and every step in that direction will improve their chances of success.

So if you truly want to manage your weight, you must program your environment in every possible way to avoid difficult foods, binge foods, and reminders to eat. In doing so, you can meaningfully influence and control your eating behavior.

PERSONAL ENVIRONMENT AUDIT

Let's begin this process by auditing your environment and your level of exposure to food and to reminders of food. What I want you to do here is to take a critical and probing inventory of the food in your home, office, your car, anywhere you stash food, encounter food, or are exposed to reminders of food, in order to see exactly how problematic your world is. Without this critical review, you will continue to be influenced by situations in your environment that are setting you up for disaster. In answering the questions below, circle either *yes* or *no* for each of the twenty questions. Unless you are 100 percent honest in your inventory, you are doing yourself no good.

1. Do you keep lots of junk food in your house?   **Yes/No**

2. Do you store food in your house in plain sight?   **Yes/No**

3. Do you have candy-filled dishes and/or bowls of nuts in your house?   **Yes/No**

4. Do you store food in rooms of your house other than your kitchen?   **Yes/No**

5. Does your desk drawer look like a convenience store?   **Yes/No**

6. Do you keep food stashed in your glove compartment or purse?   **Yes/No**

7. Do you routinely prepare family-style meals served on large platters?   **Yes/No**

8. Do you choose restaurants with buffets or family-size meals?   **Yes/No**

9. Do you have numerous diet books in your house?   **Yes/No**

10. Do you eat by the clock?   **Yes/No**

11. Does your daily route take you by vending machines, restaurants, bakeries, or other eateries?   **Yes/No**

12. Do you shop without a grocery list?   **Yes/No**

13. Does the presence of specific people trigger you to eat?   **Yes/No**

14. Do you prepare snacks for your kids or spouse?   **Yes/No**

15. Are you the only one who cleans up the kitchen after a meal?   **Yes/No**

16. Do you keep fattening foods easily accessible?   **Yes/No**

17. Do you buy fattening foods in large packages?   **Yes/No**

18. Do you buy extra-large bags of easy-to-eat processed foods (such as chips, candy, or cookies)?   **Yes/No**

19. Are you reluctant to throw out fattening leftovers?   **Yes/No**

20. Do you plan what you will eat prior to going to a restaurant?   **Yes/No**

SCORING AND INTERPRETATION

For every "yes" answer, assign one point, and add up your total. Realistically, any score higher than two indicates that your environment is a standing invitation to eat. If your total score is ten or higher, your environment is riddled with problems. Food is everywhere you turn—your house, your car, your office. It's tough to exercise control when food and reminders of food are so prevalent in your life. Yours is a temptation-rich environment, for sure, but remember, it is the environment over which you have the most control.

THE POWER OF CUES

For this key to fit the lock, that is, get you through the door of external control, I must first talk to you about the "cues" operating in your environment and how they're standing in your way to positive change. In theatrical terms, a cue is a signal to a performer to recite a line or begin a certain action. Similarly, eating cues—which are basically reminders of food—trigger your decision to eat. If you prefer the "shrink" term for cues, they are stimuli that elicit your response, and that response is to eat. Most overweight people are more vulnerable to cues than are their thin counterparts—much research bears this out.

Eating cues are either *external* or *internal*. Some internal cues are physical; that is, they're signs of true biological hunger, brought on by specific responses that go on inside your body because it demands nourishment. Some of the main internal cues for eating include stomach contractions (the growling or gurgling you experience when your stomach is empty) and a physical weakness brought on by low levels of blood sugar, the major fuel used to supply your body's energy needs. These cues arise from honest-to-goodness hunger. Hunger is, of course, a very basic motivator guiding your food choices and certainly one that is essential to your very survival.

If these were your only internal cues for eating, however, you'd probably be slender and fit because you'd eat only when truly hungry and stop when full. But many people who are overweight don't recognize when they are physiologically hungry, and instead eat according to other types of internal cues, such as painful emotions, boredom, depression, or unchecked stress. These cues are entirely psychological, rather than physiological. The desire for food comes not from your stomach, but from your head.

Let's move on to external cues. These are triggers that exist and operate in your environment, and they powerfully stimulate your urge to eat, whether you are physically hungry or not. As I've just said, if you are overweight, you typically fail to respond to biological internal cues—you *literally do not know when you are physiologically hungry*—but instead you're highly inclined to eat in response to external cues. Examples of external cues include:

- Sight of food

- Passage of time (you eat according to the clock)

- Vending machines

- Aroma of food

- Flavor of food (sugary or salty foods, in particular, have an addictive appeal)

- Watching television

- Certain locations in your house

- Being in your car

- Your office

- The route you take to or from work

- Restaurants and drive-throughs

- Watching people eat

- Being offered food

- Vacations

- Parties

- Food advertisements

- Recipes in magazines or books

Sometimes these cues scream pretty loud, catching you completely off guard. You immediately start thinking about food and want to start eating. Every time you even think about food, your body starts reacting at a physiological level to heighten your desire to eat. One of these reactions occurs within your mouth: you begin to salivate. You experience a physiological change in your mouth, and you want to eat.

Scientists also believe that another reaction is triggered, one that comes about deep within your body, at the hormonal level. Suppose you're standing in front of a bakery, drooling over a banana cream pie in the window. In response to the sight of that pie, your body begins to churn out more of the hormone *insulin*. Even if you don't eat a single morsel of pie, insulin begins to do a couple of its regular jobs. For one thing, it accelerates the intake of fat into cells for storage (yes, just looking at food may make you fat!). Second, insulin reduces levels of blood sugar in your body, which it ordinarily does after you've eaten, in order to move that blood sugar into your cells for energy. This creates a state of low blood sugar that leads to hunger.

Astonishing, isn't it? Thoughts about food, triggered by a cue, have the power to elicit dramatic physiological reactions. There is a very substantive association at work here. The cues in your environment will arouse your hunger in a big way, whether you need to eat or not, and they may even activate fat-storing processes. If you're constantly bombarded by external, environmental cues, then the physiology that simultaneously occurs will work against you.

Please recognize too, that much of this bombardment comes from the food industry, which includes companies and restaurants that produce, sell, and serve food and beverages. This industry has capitalized on powerful flavor cues by developing an ever-increasing array of high-fat, sugary, salty foods with addictive appeal and by encouraging you—through advertising—to eat more of them. The imperatives of the food industry, in order to drive profits and make shareholders happy, are to lace foods with sugar, salt, and fat, and to make these foods convenient and readily accessible so that as a food-buying public, we'll eat them quicker than God can get news. Giving our power away and letting the food industry make our choices for us has become a growth industry—an $800 billion industry at last count, in fact. It should come as no surprise to you that millions of people look to the food industry to make their choices for them, from breakfast all the way to late-night snacking, a job that this industry is more than happy to perform. As food buyers, we've yielded our power to choose. Consider the proof: if you are the average, typical American, you consume roughly 158 pounds of sugar a year, in the form of pure sugar, corn sweeteners, honey, maple syrup, other edible syrups found in soft drinks, sweets, commercially baked foods, and other processed foods. You are also eating, on average, 63 pounds of added fat a year (that's double what people ate in the early twentieth century) from the butter on your bread to fats and oils used in fried foods and commercially prepared cookies and pastries.

If you regularly watch television—the most widely used advertising medium—you are being bombarded with messages that tell you what to eat, where to eat, when to eat, and why to eat. (I do not want to let it go unnoticed that now there is an entire network devoted to food, and to food only.)

Not by accident, the most heavily advertised foods are the ones most responsible for the obesity epidemic: fast foods (fast-food restaurants plunk down most of their ad budget on TV commercials), snacks, candy, prepared convenience foods, soft drinks, and alcoholic beverages. You are urged to eat them in your car, at parties, at sporting events, in restaurants, at movie theaters—practically everywhere except your dining room table. To make matters worse, a lot of you are eating them in front of your TV—a behavior that has been shown to pack on 14 pounds a year.

Food advertising sells you food emotionally—have you noticed? Eat more food and it will bring more fun, happiness, belonging— even love, to the point of sometimes suggesting that food will help you attract someone of the opposite sex. By appealing to other human motivations, ad campaigns like "Join the Pepsi Generation" play on your need for acceptance and belonging, the emotional desire to be part of a family, an organization, or a peer group. Beer ads like "Grab all the gusto you can" tug on your inner need for self-worth, telling you beer will help you realize your full potential as a person. The more your internally defined self-worth is lacking, the more vulnerable you are to this type of external cue. In short, if you aren't squared away within yourself, messages like these can get to you from the outside. You'll cave in to eating and drinking stuff you certainly don't need.

The food industry is pushing a "make eating fast" agenda, as well.

Since 1972, the number of fast-food restaurants in the United States has doubled, hawking high-fat, high-calorie, nutritionally weak foods to millions of consumers only too willing to gobble them up. Burger King alone sells 4 million Whoppers a day!

It is a fact of modern life that you find fast-food restaurants everywhere these days, but their latest encroachment is in the most unlikely and surprising place of all: hospitals. I recently read a national news item reporting that more than a third of America's sixteen top hospitals now have regional or national fast-food franchises on their premises. Talk about mixed messages: we're obese because we eat too much fast food but while we're in the hospital being treated for obesity-related diseases, we can eat more fast foods. I don't know what gives, or where it all ends, but somebody's lost too many balls in the high weeds.

Along with our waistlines, portion sizes in prepackaged ready-to-eat foods and at restaurants are getting bigger and bigger. This is in part because, as consumers we value a greater quantity of food and drink for a lower price—a "value" that the food industry is more than willing to provide. A good example is the soft drink. Where once the 12-ounce soft drink can was the norm, it has now been displaced by the 20-ounce bottle, sold in vending machines, at convenience stores, and elsewhere. As for food, go to any fast-food restaurant and on the menu you will find not only large, medium, and small, but "super-size," "king-size," "queen-size," "monster meals," and "biggie" items.

You need to go on the alert here, that you and your family are being targeted by these billion-bucks industries. I'm calling on you to "move the target"—that's you—so that you miss their aim. Move the target by not buying into this stuff. If you continue to let the food industry make your choices for you, then you're setting yourself up for more years of living in the same state of continuous chaos. It's about you deciding whether you are going to be the bull's-eye for the rest of your life, waiting to get hit by the arrow. You control what you buy or don't buy, you control where you decide to eat, and what you decide to eat when you get there. Like it or not, a lot of cause and effect is in your hands. The greater the knowledge you have about what's going on in the world around you, the more power you have to control the outcomes in your life.

CUE ELIMINATION

Clearly, cues govern your behavior in powerful ways—which is why you have to eliminate as many of them as you reasonably can from your own environment, and make choices to avoid them. When you rid your world of cues, making small but meaningful adjustments to your lifestyle, you powerfully program yourself against the possibility of weight gain.

If you have any doubts about the power of cue elimination on your behavior, think about anti-smoking reforms. State laws restricting smoking in public places; smoke-free office policies; cigarette taxes; and restrictions on tobacco advertising and promotion have been enacted that have made smoking very difficult. And according to 2002 figures from the American Lung Association, smoking has been significantly on the decline for the past forty years. Even cases of lung cancer have been steadily decreasing, particularly among men, as people smoke fewer cigarettes a day or quit altogether. In states where there is vigorous enforcement of tobacco control, fewer young adults are opting to smoke, although elsewhere tobacco use is unfortunately increasing among this population. What these trends suggest is that the removal of opportunities to smoke, and the removal of messages to smoke, have helped lessen a highly destructive behavior—one that is responsible for one in five deaths in the United States—and have done so in a dramatic way.

I'm making such a big deal out of this because I know that if you remove access and opportunity to behave in a negative manner, you are less likely to engage in that behavior. Granted, unlike tobacco, alcohol, and drugs, food is a substance from which you cannot totally abstain. But you are not powerless against it.

So if you want to lose weight, you must make your environment as free and as safe from fattening foods as possible, because wherever there's food that's easy to eat, you'll eat it. Programming your environment in this way will produce near-automatic changes in your behavior, making it totally unnecessary to rely on willpower. Sure, willpower helps you build up a short-lived burst of energy that will lead to some temporary changes, but it is never going to be enough. When willpower fades, you'll resume your old patterns of eating and coping. You'll eat everything that isn't moving. You'll lose days and weeks of hard-won control. And you'll regain your weight. Programming, on the other hand, moves you out of the repetitious rut of bad habits and gets you into the groove of permanent weight control.

For example, if you always grab a handful of candy from the candy dish next to your sofa, it doesn't make sense to battle the fickle emotion of willpower in order to resist the urge to eat it. The best way to deal with that candy is to empty the dish and get rid of the stuff. You can't eat what's not there, so pretty soon your candy-eating habit will no longer have you in its clutches. Failure-proofing your environment doesn't involve any big inner struggle, either. All it involves is removing fattening impulse foods from your line of sight.

In my own life, I've experienced how dramatically effective programming can be. I am invariably hungry when I come home at the end of the day. For the longest time, I would enter the house through a door that led me through the kitchen. I would tell myself repeatedly that I wasn't going to snack before dinner. Sometimes the emotion of willpower would carry me, sometimes it wouldn't. As I cruised through the kitchen, the environment was full of temptation, and I'd start grabbing junk foods, right and left. Maybe they were cookies on a platter one day, a chocolate cake the next, or some other food I would quickly consume. It was not unusual for me to wolf down anywhere between 1,500 and 10,000 calories in one sitting ("standing" would be a more apt description), shower, then sit down for a full dinner. Essentially, I was eating twice.

To program myself for success, I just started entering the house through another door that did not take me through the kitchen. The route I took had no opportunities for failure, and I got past the habitual, reactive snacking that had plagued me. By the time I sat down for dinner, I was eating only once, instead of a couple of times. Believe me, this method is a lot more pleasant, and effective, than having to muster up willpower.

The significance of programming is that it recognizes that your life is full of temptations to overeat and opportunities to fail at weight control. But when you learn to reprogram all the wrong things you have been doing, you will discover that it is so much easier to lose weight because your life will no longer revolve around food.

The best and most effective way to deal with cues is to wipe them from your environment or lessen your exposure to them. If you never see cookies, you will lose your cookie-eating desires, and cookies will eventually become less tempting. Further, if you replace those cookies with apples, oranges, or some other healthy snack food, a new preference is developed. Each time you choose the healthier substitute, that preference gets stronger and more appetizing. You already know this yourself if there was ever a time in your life when you used to drink whole milk, and then for whatever reason you switched to drinking skim milk. At first, you found the taste of skim milk bland and watery, but you just kept on drinking it. Eventually, you began to enjoy skim milk, and in fact, now you actually find that drinking whole milk is quite objectionable because it tastes too heavy and rich.

I don't want to just blow by this. Decreasing access and exposure to foods is a big deal, it works, and it has been scientifically verified to work too. In numerous experiments, investigators have shown that a person's choice will shift from high-calorie, high-fat snack foods to healthy foods when it becomes difficult to obtain the snack foods but easier to get fruits, vegetables, and other more nutritious snacks. This research into what investigators call *choice shift* acknowledges—and proves—some commonsense wisdom: you'll eat what's available, you can't eat what's not there, and you won't eat what you don't buy. It also shows that after a period of new eating behavior, you may not desire any snack food other than foods like plump, juicy fruits, or delicious, satisfying vegetables.

ACTION STEPS THROUGH THE DOOR TO EXTERNAL CONTROL

What I'm now challenging you to do is reduce the availability of fattening foods so that your own food choices will shift to healthier and more nutritious foods. I want you to make sure that your exposure to high-calorie, high-fat junk foods, and the cues to eat them, are greatly reduced in your environment. There is no room here for cutting corners or rationalizing the maintenance of any of these cues in your life. You are dealing with environmental influences that you set up through the choices you made. I also want to challenge you to listen to internal cues signaling true physical hunger—and eat in response to those, rather than to external cues. Here are the steps.

STEP ONE: MAKE YOUR ENVIRONMENT SAFE

Thinking about the important work you completed in the Personal Environment Audit, what I'd like you to do is comb your pantry, your refrigerator, your closet, your drawers—wherever you store food—and see what you can throw away, or at least minimize in terms of your exposure to it. It is certainly not unreasonable to rid your environment of any of the following:

- Cookies, candy, and any high-calorie, sweetened snack foods

- Salty foods such as potato chips, pretzels, taco chips, nuts, and other packaged munchies

- Sweet rolls and doughnuts

- White bread, white rolls, white buns

- Crackers

- Cold cuts

- Ice cream and high-sugar frozen desserts

- Quick-fix prepared foods such as pizza, fried entrees and dinners, microwavable sandwiches (If the food in question requires no preparation, throw it out or at least store it out of sight.)

- Syrups, jams, and jellies

- High-fat spreads, peanut butter, and dips

- Sugared soft drinks and beverages

- Alcoholic beverages

- Any food that can be classified as junk food

- Any food that you habitually binge on

I do believe that eventually many of you will be able to develop a healthy relationship with food and will not have to deprive yourself or be afraid of certain foods. But for the time being, toss this stuff out, feed it to the garbage disposal, take it to the Dumpster, or a least get it out of your sight. Do this now, do this right away, so that it is impossible for you to fail. Begin today to reprogram your environment and set yourself up for success.

Okay, I suspect that right now you are thinking, "Well, that sounds fine and good, but there are foods I need to keep around for my kids. They aren't fat. Why should they suffer?"

Trust me, I understand your concern, having experienced it in my own family. Robin and I have a very active, athletic sixteen-year-old son, Jordan, who in addition to the healthy stuff we eat at our house also likes pizza, brownies, potato chips, and all the rest. Seriously—what teenager doesn't? For those of you in the same boat, there are solutions if you have to keep these foods around. What we do at home, for example, is designate a specific cabinet in our kitchen for Jordan's foods and snacks. That's his territory, and it's off-limits to anyone but him. We don't go pecking around his food.

Barbara, a woman who has been using the seven keys to lose 80 pounds, asked her 6-foot, 5-inch husband to store fattening food in the top shelf of a kitchen cabinet that she, at 5 feet, 3 inches, could not possibly reach without going to considerable trouble. "After a few days, I honestly forgot about that food, since I've never used that cabinet, not even for dishes," she told me. "Out of sight, out of mind has been a godsend for me."

Then there is Taylor, a single mom on the road to losing 35 pounds using the seven keys. She had wanted desperately to lose weight in order to be attractive and start dating again, but she just could not keep the weight off for any reasonable length of time.

Until using the keys, Taylor kept a lot of cookies around for her two children, but not only that, she kept them in plain view, in a large cookie jar. She admitted to overindulging in cookies herself "because they were there," and these indulgences led to full-blown binges and their resultant weight gain. Ultimately, what Taylor decided to do was empty the cookie jar and put pet treats in it instead. As for the cookies, she stored them in an empty drawer in a corner of her kitchen that she hardly ever uses, or even goes near.

Another way to decrease your exposure to foods you buy for your kids is to purchase these foods in smaller packages. Rather than get a jumbo sack of chips that you're likely to scarf down in one sitting, why not buy smaller single-serving sizes? With this approach, you've got automatic portion control. Yes, it's costlier, money-wise, to buy food in single-serving packages rather than in the economy sizes, but far less costly to your weight and to your health.

But I pause here to issue a critical caveat: you do need to monitor what your child eats or does not eat. Too much unhealthy food can actually harm your children's health and pave the way to childhood obesity, and with it a slew of medical and emotional problems. The rate of childhood obesity in this country is reeling out of control. If you don't think so, just take a trip to the nearest fast-food restaurant in your neighborhood and observe the roly-poly jowls and balloon tummies on grade school kids and teens lining up for super-size meals.

As a parent, you are the person who is the food buyer and food preparer in your family. That means you are accountable for your kids' health and well-being while they are under your care. Start setting the right example by buying healthy snacks and serving nutritious meals for your household. Your kids reflect what they see in you, and they will take your example far more seriously than they will take your advice. You are their role model; be a healthy, responsible one.

There are two other related concerns we need to address right away. First, are you preparing or purchasing foods that you say your kids like, but secretly, they're your favorite binge foods? Maybe you're baking peanut butter cookies because you crave them, not because they're your kids' favorite cookies. Maybe those taco chips stashed in the cupboard are for your late-night snacking, and not really an after-school snack for your son or daughter. Don't con yourself here. If you feel you must keep certain foods on hand for your family, make sure that these are foods your kids or spouse really like—not foods you want. I'm calling your attention to this because honesty here is absolutely fundamental to managing and programming your environment for success.

You can con yourself in another way too: by telling yourself that if you get rid of all the goodies your kids like, they will think you don't love them anymore. Hold it, let's take an intermission to examine the faulty logic at work here: you believe you are loving your children with food, when in fact you are poisoning them with too much junk food that will someday make them physically sick and obese. Feeding your family with nutritionally weak food is toxic in its eventual outcome. How dumb is that? Look at it this way: the sooner you interrupt your family's habit of eating junk food, the easier it will be to establish new, healthier, more productive behaviors in their lives. Consider the advantages these healthy actions afford you in nurturing your family. You will be healthier and in better shape, and so will they. That is an incredible display of love.

STEP TWO: BEGIN THE PROCESS OF CHOICE SHIFT

This step is simple and straightforward—more commonsense than anything else. It stands to reason that as you remove junk foods from your environment or place them out of sight, you must replace them with better foods so that your food choices will naturally and eventually shift to healthier alternatives. Begin to stock your kitchen with:

- Fruits

- Vegetables

- Whole grains

- Lean meats

- Low-fat milk products (milk, yogurt, hard and soft cheeses, etc.)

- Low-fat or fat-free foods or snacks

- Sugar-free beverages

Remember what the principle of choice shift says: your taste preferences will shift to healthier, more nourishing foods if you give yourself every chance to break from the old and come in with the new.

STEP THREE: PRACTICE SMART SHOPPING

This step addresses one of the most temptation-rich environments you will ever encounter—the grocery store, where there are more than 50,000 food items, all packaged attractively and positioned strategically on the shelves to get you to buy them. Step Three helps brace you against their allure, so that you can exert an astonishing level of control in this environment. Make it a point to:

- Shop from a grocery list prepared when you are not hungry or stressed out.

- Determine exactly what you need for a particular period of time, and don't overbuy.

- Stick to the outer aisles where the fresh, additive-free foods are located, when you are grocery shopping. There's a logical reason for this placement: fresh foods require more frequent restocking and therefore must be situated as close to the outside shipping docks and stock rooms as possible.

- Never go grocery shopping when you're hungry. The entire store, from the food aisles to the checkout line, can tempt you to buy foods that you neither want nor need.

- Assign someone else in your family the job of grocery shopping on occasion in order to limit your exposure to food.

STEP FOUR: MAKE CHANGES AWAY FROM HOME

As a part of failure-proofing your environment, you must have particular plans in place for handling what could be some of the weakest spots in your efforts, such as eating out, eating away from home, or eating too much while on vacation.

Whatever your trouble spot is—and I'm sure you already know it—you need to have some strategies in place to overcome these prominent weaknesses because there are going to be situations that will arise when you will be faced with challenges and temptations. For many of you, eating away from home is problematic. The key is to take some time to plan for those situations and identify those things that could and should be the focus of your management efforts. When you are dining out, for example, choose a restaurant that offers a variety of foods so that you can choose healthier menu items. Plan ahead of time what you will order. When you get there, be assertive with the waitstaff; tell your server you want your food prepared without fats, oils, or sauces.

At parties, get in the habit of passing up the fattening food and opting for healthier choices instead. Choose smaller portions, and ask for a diet soda or club soda in lieu of an alcoholic drink. Stand away from the food, and focus on people and conversations, rather than on food.

Vacations can be difficult, but try to exert the same control in your choices that you would at home. If you are flying, you don't have to settle for the typical airline food. Simply call the airline ahead of time and request a low-calorie meal. You can do this practically anywhere, even on cruises, as long as you give the food preparation personnel plenty of notice. Compensate for eating calorie-dense foods by staying active while on vacation. If the circumstances are such that you simply cannot control your choices, take it easy, and eat smaller portions.

Bottom line: there's no good reason for you to experience any backsliding when you have a strategy in place to handle it. When these situations arise, as you know they will, you won't panic and start eating everything in sight. You will simply say to yourself, "This is the very thing I knew would happen, and I know how to deal with it. I won't panic, and I won't give in just because I am encountering normal challenges of day-to-day life. I am in control."

Before leaving our discussion of how to fat-proof your environment, let's get real about one additional dimension of your life. Sometimes the most problematic aspect of the environment in which you interact is not your home, but your place of employment. You might be in a job that pays you pretty well, but here's the deal: it is contributing to your obesity. If you work in a restaurant or grocery store, for example, you're surrounded by food day in and day out, and this assault of food cues is creating disaster in your life.

I recall a young man named Stephen from one of my seminars who absolutely craved desserts. Although he managed his weight fairly well while attending college, every summer he would take a job at a restaurant, working as a waiter at night and doing food prep during the day. The food prep part of the job involved slicing cheesecakes and preparing ice cream parfaits. The trouble was, before long

Stephen was gobbling down more cheesecakes and parfaits than he was preparing. Being around these fattening foods crushed his resolve, and his weight began to pile back on, and with it, the guilt over eating fattening foods. The fact that Stephen worked to earn money during the summer was admirable and honorable, but the problem was the interfering nature of his job choice. Because he was especially vulnerable to food cues, he should not have worked in a restaurant.

Look at it this way: if you were an alcoholic, would you apply for a job as a bartender? How dumb is that? I don't really have to tell you that if you are chronically overweight, you should not work in the food business, do I? It comes back to the fact that your job may be a toxic, high-risk situation, one that is producing negative momentum. The hard, cold reality is that you might have to start looking for employment in another field. If you value your health and your life, dig down and find the courage to change your job or career. I know this is scary, but stop denying yourself the chance of getting what you truly want. You deserve it and you are worth it.

STEP FIVE: DO A CLOSET CLEANUP.

This final step challenges you to make a no-turning-back commitment to losing weight and keeping it off. It is very specific in its instructions: do a "closet cleanup" in which you throw away your "fat wardrobe," or donate it to charity, so that you have no oversize clothes to return to, ever. Doing so builds another level of accountability into your life that will help you stay the course.

Let me tell you why this is so important: if you hang on to your larger-size clothes, this means that subconsciously you're expecting to fit back into them someday. You're clinging to a "fat" lifestyle, and psychologically to a "fat" mind-set. You're telling yourself, "This won't work either." If those clothes stay in your closet, you are committing to failure. By contrast, having no fat clothes to return to is just one more motivating factor that will help you reach—and remain at—your ideal weight.

Throw away your elastic pants; full-figure fashions; oversize housedresses; muu muus; "big men's" clothes; and all expandable clothes (don't leave yourself any "wiggle" room). As you work your way down in weight, rid your closet of clothes that are too big for you. Women, if you wear a size 18 and you once wore a size 24, throw out any clothes that are larger than a size 18, so that you have no larger sizes to return to. Guys, if you used to fit into size 80-waist pants and you've trimmed your belly down to a size 46, clear your closet of anything greater than your size 46s. You must do what is required here if you expect to succeed.

Should your smaller-size clothes ever start feeling snug again, you are out of luck. You can't wear your size 18s or 24s anymore because you no longer own a wardrobe in those sizes. You won't have anything to wear, and you would never think of running errands or going to work naked. This means it's time for a reality check: you've let things slide, and you're gaining weight again. Don't go out and buy another whole fat wardrobe; get back on track.

There should be no regression or retreat to what you have always done before, or to what you have always been. Have the willingness and courage to throw off your past, go after your weight-control goals, and pursue a life that is defined as healthy and fit.

When you revamp your environment using the steps I've discussed, you'll discover that weight control is so much easier than ever using a whit of willpower (which is impossible anyway). Removing access to and availability of fattening food will succeed like nothing you've ever tried before. It's one of the easiest ways to lose excess pounds. Yes, it does require some effort on your part. But keep at it, because these are vital real-life steps that will help you lose pounds, stay fit, and feel happier for life.

7

Key Four:
Mastery Over Food
and Impulse Eating
Unlock the Door to Habit Control

A nail is driven out by another nail. Habit is overcome by habit.
—DESIDERIUS ERASMUS

KEY #4: MASTERY OVER FOOD AND IMPULSE EATING.

You can behave your way to a healthy, fit body. If you change what you do, and you change the payoffs or rewards that you get, you move closer to permanent weight loss.

This key unlocks the door to *habit control*, a brand new, healthier relationship with food, where food is no longer at the center of your universe. It's all about disciplining yourself toward healthy behavior and creating the healthy results that flow from it. When you choose the behavior, you choose the consequences. Using this key will require examining your bad habits—and why they persist—and deciding that isn't what you want anymore. Then you can start behaving in ways that make you feel really good about yourself.

Once you realize the extent to which eating behavior is ruled by habit, you will be amazed. Some examples: Jennifer comes home from work, makes a beeline to the refrigerator, cruises its contents, and samples bits and pieces of food as if they were selections on a smorgasbord. A meatball here, a slice of cheese there. What she does not realize is that this habitual snacking adds up to 300 additional calories a day—calories she doesn't count or even think about as she grazes on the goodies in her fridge. If she continues at that rate, she'll gain 25 extra pounds this year. She doesn't understand why it is so hard to lose weight.

For Tim, who habitually eats in front of the TV, the start of the 6 o'clock news is like a dinner bell, and like Pavlov's dogs, which were conditioned to associate food with the ringing of a bell, he starts salivating and feeling the urge to eat. He eats dinner while watching the news, but afterwards has no idea how much he ate. Tim is 30 pounds heavier than he was five years ago, but hasn't a clue as to why.

Teresa would love to weigh 115 pounds again. But today she tips the scales at 200 pounds. She cares about her personal appearance and dresses and grooms herself immaculately, hoping that this will compensate for her unsightly pounds. But most nights, after her kids have gone to sleep, Teresa takes a large bag of potato chips to bed with her and reads a book while munching away.

As you read about Jennifer, Tim, and Teresa, did you notice a pattern in their eating behavior that is present in your own? All were eating in places other than the dining room table. All were eating in an unconscious manner, ignoring the experience of eating, eating simply because of reflex, or concentrating on other things while consuming the food. Because their behavior had become almost automatic, they had stopped paying attention to what they were eating, how much they were eating, where they were eating, and what the real consequences of their eating behavior were.

Like Jennifer, Tim, and Teresa, much of what you do is habitual—counterproductive patterns that you do over and over, time and time again. With most types of habitual behavior, including overeating, you started it for one reason, but continued it for another. There is a good example in gambling. A person tries gambling one day for the fun of it, then continues to gamble, now in an attempt to win money. He gambles again and again, repeating the behavior, and eventually he gets hooked on it.

What about you? Did you start bingeing or overeating for one reason, such as a betrayal, a job loss, an illness, some personal tragedy, and you've kept on doing it as a matter of habit? Your pounds came on quickly, but the trouble is, they stayed, because now you are overeating habitually, whether you are hungry or not.

Are there eating situations in your life in which you seem to go on automatic pilot, not really thinking about food as you eat it? When eating behavior becomes automatic, you stop paying attention to or evaluating the cause-and-effect relationships in the behavior. But the truth is, if you stop this pattern of mindless, automatic eating, you can slash your caloric consumption significantly and begin to regain control of your weight, almost effortlessly.

BEHAVIORAL AUDIT

As our first move in this direction, please take this brief test in order to gain insight into the ways you act and interact with food. This assessment will help you isolate which behaviors are generating the worst results, and give you a self-awareness that will help you on your way to permanent weight loss and control. Consider carefully each question below, and mark the answer that best describes your individual behavior. Answer all fifteen questions.

1. You eat large amounts of food very fast in a short amount of time:
   a. Rarely.
   b. Sometimes, when you are rushed.
   c. Most of the time, especially during the day.
   d. Usually all the time; it is a habit.

2. You eat dessert or leftovers, even if you feel full after a meal:
   a. Rarely.
   b. Sometimes, especially when you feel like you have to for social reasons.
   c. Most of the time, just because you like the taste.
   d. Usually all the time; it is a habit.

3. You sneak food:
   a. Rarely.
   b. Sometimes, especially when you are bored or stressed.
   c. Most of the time, sometimes out of spite.
   d. Usually all the time; it is a habit.

4. During a normal day, you feel the urge to eat:
   a. Only when it is mealtime.
   b. Occasionally, especially when my day is stressful.
   c. Most of the time, especially when someone talks about it.
   d. All the time; you are constantly thinking about food.

5. Usually the duration of your meals is:
   a. 30 to 45 minutes.
   b. 15 to 30 minutes.
   c. 5 to 15 minutes.
   d. You really do not take time for meals; you grab food when you can.

6. When a craving or urge to overeat a certain food comes over you, you usually:
   a. Dismiss the thought because it will pass.
   b. Purposely engage in a nonfood-related activity or pastime.
   c. Use a substitute food.
   d. Give in to it.

7. You leave food on your plate:
   a. Usually.
   b. Occasionally.
   c. Once in a while.
   d. Never.

8. You typically eat large meals even if you are not hungry:
   a. Rarely.
   b. Usually at a friend or family member's insistence.
   c. When you are depressed or anxious.
   d. Frequently.

9. You watch TV or engage in other activities while eating:
   a. Rarely.
   b. Occasionally.
   c. More often than not.
   d. Most of the time.

10. How many rooms of your home do you eat in?
    a. One.
    b. Two.
    c. Three.
    d. More than three.

11. How many of your pleasurable activities center around food?
    a. 0 to 25 percent.
    b. 26 to 50 percent.
    c. 51 to 75 percent.
    d. 76 to 100 percent.

12. How often do you engage in behaviors such as binge eating or nighttime eating?
    a. Never.
    b. Some of the time.
    c. Often.
    d. Frequently.

13. With your meals, your portions are usually:
    a. Small.
    b. Medium.
    c. Large.
    d. Large; plus you habitually have second helpings.

14. When you feel tired, you:
    a. Lie down to rest, or take a nap.
    b. Do nothing and hope it will pass.
    c. Have a snack.
    d. Binge on high-calorie, sugary foods.

15. When you have a meal, you thoroughly chew your food and savor each bite:
    a. Always.
    b. Occasionally.
    c. Seldom.
    d. Never; it goes down too fast.

SCORING

For each "a" you checked, give yourself a credit of 1; for each "b" you checked, give yourself no credit (0); for each "c," give yourself one negative credit (−1); and for each "d," give yourself two negative credits (−2). Adding up each item for all 15 items, you should have a total in a range from +15 to −30.

Interpretation

+5 to +15: A score in this range means that generally you behave in ways that are healthy and help you control your weight. You may have some behavioral habits that are changeworthy, however. You can identify these by reviewing answers in which you circled "c" or "d." Keep reading and doing the important work found in this key, and you'll learn successful steps to help you take off pounds and better control your weight.

−5 to +4: This range suggests that you are demonstrating a pattern of behavior that, in a number of instances, runs counter to good weight control. You'll learn some remarkable tools here to help you get better results.

−15 to −6: A score in this range indicates that your behavioral habits are perpetuating your weight problem. You need to pay closer attention to your food and eating behaviors in order to make the substantial changes needed. Accept this challenge and do not give up on yourself.

−30 to −16: If your score falls in this range, you will have to start making significant turnabouts in how you interact with food if you want to experience the weight loss and control that come from healthy food and eating behaviors. Make a concerted effort to initiate change immediately.

Okay, now that you've taken this audit, we're ready to work on specific behaviors that have been your downfall in the past. That means you'll be behaving your way toward your weight loss goals. Don't get this mixed up with the less genuine technique of "fake it till you make it." You won't be faking successful behaviors in any way. You genuinely do want a healthy weight you can maintain. If you begin to behave in ways that reflect and define your weight-control priorities, then you'll start enjoying the consequences of that behavior. You'll begin to feel lighter, stronger, and more alive than ever.

If you were honest in your answers to the Behavioral Audit you took early on, then you already know a great deal about the problematic behaviors impacting your weight. Depending on your responses to individual questions on the audit, these behaviors may include:

- Eating too fast or too much

- Eating leftovers or dessert

- Eating sweet, high-fat food as a matter of habit

- Sneaking food

- Giving in to urges or cues to overeat

- Cleaning your plate most of the time

- Eating in locations other than at your kitchen or dining room tables

- Centering activities around food

- Bingeing

- Nighttime eating

Study this list very carefully and look back over your answers on the audit you took. In completing this inventory, you probably identified some rather glaring behaviors. And because you can't change what you don't acknowledge, you've taken some huge steps toward lifelong weight control. What I want you to see now is that these behaviors can lead directly to the pounds you're packing. They're the price you pay for the shape you're in.

To bring this point into sharper focus, please take a good look at the table below. It is what I call my "hit list" of weight-gaining behaviors—things you do that really stack up, calorie-wise and pound-wise. Also, note in the fourth column how much weight you can gain over the course of one year unless you stop these eating behaviors. (I

TABLE 3. HIT LIST OF WEIGHT-GAINING BEHAVIORS

Eating Behavior	Weekly Caloric Cost	Annual Caloric Cost	Potential Weight Gain Per Year (3,500 extra calories = 1 pound)
Eating second helpings (200 calories per helping) three times a week	600 extra calories a week	31,200 extra calories a year	9 pounds
Habitual overeating, every day, 380 extra calories a day	2,660 extra calories a week	138,320 extra calories a year	40 pounds*
Eating a super-size bagel (4½" diameter, 323 calories), three times a week, rather than having a small bagel (3" diameter, 156 calories)	500 extra calories a week	26,000 extra calories a year	8 pounds*
Eating Big Macs (or equivalent, 570 calories) twice a week, rather than choosing a small-size hamburger (260 calories)	620 extra calories a week	32,240 extra calories a year	9 pounds
Eating one glazed doughnut (290 calories) every day at work during your coffee break	1,450 extra calories a week	75,400 extra calories a year	21 pounds*
Drinking a cup of whole milk (150 calories) twice a day, rather than having skim milk (86 calories)	896 extra calories a week	46,600 extra calories a year	13 pounds
Drinking one regular soda a day (144 calories), rather than having a calorie-free soda	1,008 extra calories a week	52,400 extra calories a year	15 pounds
Snacking on 15 to 20 potato chips a day (150 calories)	1,050 extra calories a week	54,600 extra calories a year	16 pounds*
Eating a bowl of regular ice cream (280 calories) five times a week, rather than having a bowl of nonfat frozen yogurt (160 calories)	600 extra calories a week	31,200 extra calories a year	9 pounds
Bingeing twice a week (1,000 to 3,000 calories per binge)	2,000 to 6,000 extra calories a week	104,000 to 312,000 extra calories a year	30 to 90 pounds
Eating out at fast-food restaurants five times a week compared to having a healthy meal prepared at home (56 extra calories per fast-food meal)	280 extra calories a week	14,560 extra calories a year	4 pounds
Snacking while watching television, five hours a week (136 extra calories per snack)	680 extra calories a week	35,360 extra calories a year	10 pounds
Nighttime eating, five episodes a week (270 calories per episode)	1,350 extra calories a week	70,200 extra calories a year	20 pounds
Drinking three beers at Happy Hour once a week (146 calories per beer)	438 extra calories a week	22,776 extra calories a year	6½ pounds

The information in this chart is based on typical calorie counts of foods and beverages, as well as on scientific studies of the caloric cost of specific eating behaviors. Results may vary from person to person. Annual weight gain is based on calculating the estimated yearly caloric cost of each behavior, then dividing by 3,500 calories (the number of additional calories it takes to gain one pound).
* These figures have been rounded up.

hope your jaw drops in amazement right now!) There's a real cause-and-effect association at work here, and I want to make sure you get it.

PROBE YOUR PAYOFFS

Up until now, you may have been doing these things, going about your day, with little or no appreciation of their gravity or impact. But with enough time and repetition, these behaviors create results, and those results are weight gain. That is both the good news and the bad news. You're behaving in ways that are making you bigger and rounder, but you can also stop behaving like that and see your waist again. It's under your control. So if you're serious about losing weight, you'll work at stopping the behaviors that have so persistently and destructively kept you overweight and out of shape. Looking back over this table for a moment and reconsidering your answers to the Behavioral Audit, you may logically wonder: if these behaviors are making me overweight, then why do I keep doing them? Why do I keep doing something that I want to stop? Why? Why? Why? Surely no rational, logical person would purposely behave in a way that generated results that they do not want or that keep them from getting results they do want. But no matter how rational and logical you think you are, you know that is exactly what you do.

One reason is the power of the *payoff*. To understand this concept, there is a fitting illustration in the story of the celebrated bank robber, Willie Sutton, who was finally nabbed after a bank-robbing career that spanned twenty-two years. Once they had him behind bars, the police asked Sutton, "Willie, you knew you were going to get caught and sent to jail. So why did you rob banks?" Willie's often-quoted reason for his crime was, "Because that's where the money is." To Willie, the payoff for his behavior—the reason he did it—was the money he stole, but it was also what robbed him of his freedom.

One of my mantras is "People do what works." You will not maintain any behavior that is not providing you with some kind of payoff. In other words, you choose to keep doing the behavior because, at some level, it works for you. At some level it pays off for you, it generates some value for you, or you wouldn't do it. No payoff, no repetition. So based on results, since people do only what works, your behavior must work for you in some way.

To eliminate this destructive, illogical behavior, you must first understand why you do it. Knowing why you do something will help you *not* do it.

The more you understand about why you behave in ways that make you overweight, the more equipped you will be to fix your behavior. Only then can you know what buttons to push to change your behavior. This means you can start behaving in positive ways necessary to lose weight and keep it off—or just as importantly, stop behaving in ways that interfere with your weight loss goals. That being so, let's take a time-out here and deal directly with the specifics of your behavior and the payoffs you derive from it, so that you will not be controlled by these things any longer.

Do This Exercise

Please go back over your answers to the Behavioral Audit you just took. Your answers turned the floodlights on certain behaviors you need to stop in order to get your weight permanently under control. Carefully review those behaviors. Take out a pen and a piece of paper, and list the most troublesome behaviors that emerged from this audit. Then add to that list, if you can, any additional negative behaviors that are making you overweight and contributing in a toxic way to your health. Use my hit list of weight-gaining behavior to stimulate ideas.

Next comes the challenge: for each entry, identify and write down the payoff that is keeping this negative behavior alive. Because some payoffs are not so apparent, you might have to dig down deep, analyzing your situation thoroughly and considering all the possible ways you could be getting paid off without being aware of it. To help you get started, here are examples of payoffs that perpetuate weight-gaining behavior. Some of these may be contributing to your own behavior:

PLEASURE

You may overeat simply because of the sheer pleasurable sensation you get from ingesting food. It tastes good, pure and simple. For you, the sensory gratification of eating food outweighs the satisfaction of being at your ideal body weight. There's no deep, dark reason that's driving your desire for food; you just enjoy having a party in your mouth and the pleasure that comes from the event of eating food. You aren't worried about the physical, mental, or emotional cost of that party. Although it is true that people by nature are hedonistic— that is, we seek pleasure and avoid pain—you must get real about the fact that your pleasure-seeking behavior could be destroying your health and your life. If you are not willing to acknowledge the problem and what is wrong with this behavior, then you will neither lose weight, nor effect any genuine change.

PHYSIOLOGICAL CALM

When you eat, your body chemistry is altered temporarily. To assist in the process of digestion, for example, your heart pumps blood to your internal organs, and this gives you a warm, relaxed feeling. What's more, food helps your brain manufacture natural chemicals that have a soothing effect on your nervous system. There is a true physiological "high" that comes from ingesting food, and that high is a payoff you derive from eating.

EMOTIONAL RELIEF

As we have seen, food can serve a variety of purposes, far beyond simple nourishment: celebration, medication, companionship, entertainment, or avoidance of emotional resolution. Any sort of emotional high or low becomes a trigger for eating, a way of coping with shifting moods, or covering up for stress or problems you don't want to face or resolve. The downside of eating for emotional relief is that it ultimately makes you feel worse because it causes weight gain, brings on feelings of guilt, and can erode your self-esteem.

IRRATIONAL REWARDS

Far too often, we rationalize irrational behavior, and eating behavior is no exception. For example, if you have a stressful day and treat yourself to a double fudge sundae after work as a way to unwind because you "deserve it," then you're deluding yourself. That is sweet poison. This sort of payoff system, in which you reward yourself with food or overeating, is irrational, counterproductive, and cannot be a plus in any sense of the word. It undoes any good you've done to yourself and shifts into reverse any progress you've made toward your weight-loss goals. Stop justifying your behavior in this manner.

ACCEPTANCE

Maybe your payoff from overeating has to do with acceptance or belonging. And no wonder. The number one emotional need of people everywhere is the desire for acceptance: the emotional satisfaction that you are a part of a couple, family, organization, peer group, or social circle. And so you eat to be sociable and fit in. For example, if your friends and family get together frequently for huge meals, maybe you join in and start pigging out with the rest of them. The problem with this is that you're making choices out of concern for what other people might think, and the hope that by complying with what you think they want you to do, you will win their acceptance.

THE APPEAL OF IMMEDIATE VERSUS DELAYED GRATIFICATION

Our need for immediate gratification—a fast, feel-good reward right now—is a very powerful payoff. This explains why you decide to go out for beer and pizza with your friends after work rather than exercise at the gym. Eating pizza and guzzling beer with friends is fun and relaxing after work; sweating through a good workout may extend your life ten or twenty years from now. Who cares about twenty or thirty years from now? It sure feels good to eat pizza and drink beer right now. The short-term gratification you get today out-leverages the long-term costs of your self-destructive behavior.

If this is your payoff, this approach is what I call the Scarlett O'Hara school of self-management: "I will think about that tomorrow." It's an approach that disregards the long-term consequences of negative behavior on your weight, your health, your relationships, and, indeed, your overall standard of living.

SAFETY

For whatever underlying reason, remaining overweight may make you feel safe in some way. Recall the example of Sandra in Key #2, who was a victim of childhood sexual abuse. Sandra took refuge in gaining enough weight so that she felt her sexual attractiveness would be neutralized and she was therefore able to "hide" from men. Like Sandra, you may want to hide your own sexuality, and so you zip yourself up in a 100-pound parka called obesity. That way, you do not have to think about or deal with the prospects of dating, getting married, or having a family. Your weight provides you with the safety of sexual irrelevancy. Maybe it has nothing to do with sexuality, but it does have to do with a safety zone created by you to give yourself an excuse to not reach for some goal in life, because you are obese. How often have you said, "Boy, just as soon as I get this weight off of me I am going to. . . ." Give up the excuses, and lose the weight. It's time to get in the game of life.

These are examples to take into consideration as you go about identifying and writing down your own payoffs. Think about the following:

How is your weight working for you? What are your payoffs from being overweight? Is it a way of getting pleasure or emotional relief? Is food your best friend? Does your weight protect you by insulating you from other people? Do you reward yourself by overeating? Do you overeat as a way of pleasing other people or fitting into some group?

As you do this exercise, don't get discouraged. Don't give up. If you do some probing, you will discover what you are getting out of what you are doing.

Once you find the payoffs that control your behavior and make your weight what it is, you'll tell yourself: "I can see why I'm overweight. I have no reason to expect my weight to be anything other than what it is. I can see why I've gone up and down in weight so many times. I did not know why I could never lose weight before, but now I do. I've been programming myself for weight gain, not for weight loss. But no more."

The payoffs I've described for you above, and the payoffs you have listed for yourself, are not unhealthy in and of themselves. There is absolutely nothing wrong with wanting a warm feeling, desiring a sense of calm and peace, needing emotional relief, seeking love and acceptance, or finding safety. A payoff is a payoff whether it comes from food or from something else. What is unhealthy and what is destructive is how you're getting those payoffs—from food, from overeating, and from all sorts of unhealthy, inappropriate food-related behavior. I want you to have the payoffs; I just want you to stop getting them from food.

New Ways to Cope

Okay, now I'm sure you're asking yourself: "If I don't have food as a way to cope, what will I do?" Great question. It stands to reason that if food is removed as your way of coping with life, as your way of getting payoffs, you must put something else in its place, or you'll simply return to food. So what you must learn to do is replace that negative coping mechanism with more positive, constructive tools that will generate the same payoffs. From here forward, your payoffs will come from new behaviors that will make you feel good about yourself and your appearance. Keep stepping through this door with me, and you'll learn about new behaviors that will make those extra pounds come off much faster.

Introduction to Habit Control and Incompatible Behaviors

It is time to break free from your habitual dependency on food as a means of coping and take total charge of yourself. This will require weakening ingrained habits, changing self-defeating patterns, and learning how to handle your urges and impulses. You must be willing to challenge virtually every behavior pattern in your life that involves food, and be open to new ways of coping with challenges.

When you examine your own eating habits, and you discover that they are perpetuating your weight problem, then you need to get rid of them; you need to break those bad habits. "Break" is a misnomer, because we don't actually break habits. In order to eliminate one habitual behavior, you must replace it with a new behavior that is *incompatible* with the one you want to eliminate; the old, bad one will gradually lose its grip over you, since the two habits cannot co-exist. For example, it is virtually impossible to eat leftover cheesecake if you decide to take a shower instead. Taking a shower is incompatible with eating cheesecake. By the time you finish your shower and have gotten dressed, the desire to eat cheesecake has disappeared.

To fully grasp this concept, consider for a moment the struggles that alcoholics or smokers undertake in order to conquer their addictions. During those times when they are most likely to give in to the desire to drink or to smoke, you would recommend that they choose incompatible behaviors to perform instead. It is difficult for an alcoholic to drink with his buddies when he is working out in a gym, strengthening his body. Lifting weights trumps drinking. It is tough for someone to smoke while she's doing laps in the pool. Water trumps cigarettes. Weight lifting and swimming interfere with the negative behaviors, and in effect, are designed to weaken them. In the same vein, you too can powerfully change your eating behaviors by finding incompatible actions that will thwart negative outcomes.

One reason this plan of attack works so powerfully is that substituting an incompatible behavior for a bad habit takes your mind off the habit you want to weaken. There is an excellent example of this concept in the treatment of pain. Medically, it has been shown time after time that the more we concentrate on pain, the more we feel it. Focusing on something else, rather than on the pain, actually alleviates the pain.

Earlier in my career, I helped open and direct a pain clinic in which we treated people with chronic and debilitating physically-based pain. New on the job, I had organized group therapy sessions with patients who were undergoing treatment for pain. But one of my colleagues on the clinic staff cautioned me, wisely, that in group sessions, patients habitually dwell on their pain, and the more they concentrated on their pain, the more they felt it and the worse they got. And he was right. While in group therapy, all the patients thought about was their pain, and as long as they did that, in or out of therapy, they were doomed to a painful life. So instead of group therapy, we instituted an entirely different treatment strategy in which patients became purposely involved in other activities, such as playing games, taking walks, and learning relaxation techniques, rather than sitting around and wallowing in their pain.

True to what we predicted, this strategy worked. As our pain patients became absorbed in activities that distracted them from their problem, they were able to break the cycle of pain, and reduce their pain to more moderate levels—levels that could be described as manageable. With those patients who worked earnestly at restoring balance in their lives, pain diminished even more, to the point that it no longer disrupted their lives to any appreciable degree. These patients learned to create a new, alternate pattern of response to their habitual fixation, and this strongly influenced their health and their quality of life.

ACTION STEPS THROUGH THE DOOR TO HABIT CONTROL

Let's make this discussion practical by talking about your own behavior. With the steps that follow, you'll learn how to use incompatible activities to stop overeating, bingeing, and other forms of inappropriate eating; how to fight your impulses and urges; and how to change your eating style so that you feel more satisfied with less food. Together, we are about to jump-start your weight loss like never before.

STEP ONE: REPLACE BAD HABITS WITH INCOMPATIBLE ACTIONS

Using incompatible activities as substitutes for out-of-control eating is a powerful way to change your behavior. It is particularly effective if you eat habitually in response to external and internal cues—for example, the smell of food wafting from the kitchen, the hunger pangs you feel when you sink into your easy chair to watch the tube after work; or when you're suffering bouts of stress, anxiety, depression, boredom, or fatigue. Being aware of the cues that make you vulnerable to overeating helps you prepare for temptation and helps you use incompatible actions to counteract it.

If you know, for example, that at certain times of the day your temptation to overeat is the strongest, then you can schedule non-food-related activities—incompatible actions—to compete with that behavior. Or if you let yourself become so tired that you could sleep on a barbed wire fence, and you are tempted to eat enough for an army, then make it compulsory that you will take a 20-minute nap rather than raid your refrigerator. Why will this work? It will work because sleeping is incompatible with eating. So are dozens of other activities. Have you ever tried bingeing on chocolate cake while taking a bubble bath, or dancing to music while shoveling in your third bowl of cereal?

In this step, our focus will be on substituting activities that interfere with overeating, bingeing, and the other self-defeating behaviors you are trying to eliminate. There are two requirements these activities must meet. Number one, the activities you select must be available; that is, you can perform them at a moment's notice. Number two, they must compete with the action of eating. These activities form a new battery of coping tools that you can substitute for overeating. The more tools and activities you can plug into your day as coping strategies, the more likely you are to get the results you want.

You can look at it this way: when faced with the desire to overeat or binge, you are suddenly at a crossroads. If you should go right (positive choices and coping), but go left instead (poor choices or no coping at all), you're headed down a road you don't want to be on. Just as importantly, you're keeping yourself from going in the right direction. That's the kind of wrong turn that can have disastrous effects on your weight.

Okay, which activities might work for you? To help you think this through and to get you started in the right direction, I've classified activities into three broad categories: fun activities, those you do for pure enjoyment; relaxation activities, those you employ to reduce tension; and obligatory activities, those things you must do, as a matter of life maintenance, to manage your household or take care of your family. With these categories in mind, here are some examples of incompatible behaviors you might consider:

Fun:

- Pursue a favorite hobby, or take up something new you'd like to learn.

- Work in your garden.

- Play a game with your kids or your friends.

- Learn a new sport or game.

- Visit your neighbors, or talk to a friend.

- Write letters or send emails to friends or family.

- Write in your journal.

- Give yourself a manicure.

- Go to a good movie, or rent a video.

- Read your favorite magazine.

- Read a good book.

- Plan your next vacation.

- Watch a sunrise or sunset.

Relaxation:

- Do relaxation exercises. (*See Appendix A for instructions.*)

- Go for a walk, a jog, a swim, or a bike ride.

- Go to the gym and work out.

- Exercise to an exercise video.

- Dance to some upbeat music.

- Take a shower or a leisurely bath.

- Have a massage.

- Pamper yourself with a day of beauty at a day spa or salon.

- Listen to music.

- Sing along with your favorite music.

- Engage in prayer or meditation.

- Write a poem.

- Take a short nap.

- Take the day off and go on a day trip.

Obligatory:

- Do housework.

- Pay your bills.

- Balance your checkbook.

- Complete a home improvement project.

- Rearrange the furniture in a room or two.

- Wash your car.

- Clean out your closets or your drawers.

- Run errands.

- Do all the things your dentist wants you to do: brush, floss, rinse with mouthwash.

- Volunteer for a project, then follow through on your commitments.

- Take your dog for a walk.

As all of this suggests, you are going to do certain things that perhaps you haven't done before. That means the territory you're entering is uncharted, it's unknown, it's not part of your life momentum; and as a consequence, you're going to resent it at first. You're going to feel uncomfortable, with the anxiety that this discomfort brings on, because you are doing something to which you are not accustomed. It is a truth of human nature that you will want to resist things that are new and that you don't understand.

But let me get real with you: you can overcome this human truth by consciously taking on the attitude of a "willing spirit." Be willing to experiment and try new things in order to weaken your old habits.

Adopting this spirit and putting into action everything you've learned is critical to keeping your positive momentum alive. Yes, change can be painful, but it is change for the better. My dad, who had a real can-do attitude, used to say, "Successful people will do what unsuccessful people won't." If you let your judgmental, stuck-in-a-rut nature win out, you'll never, ever, get what you want. So break out of your old habitual doldrums. Climb out of your rut and look around. Give these things a try. You might be really surprised by the outcome. You don't have to like them; you just have to do them.

That said, what I now challenge you to do is compile your own list of similar activities, any of which you can substitute for inappropriate, out-of-control eating. Please write these activities down, too. Writing things down brings home the need to do them. Then tape copies of this list at any vulnerable location where you're likely to overeat—your refrigerator, your car, your television, or your desk at work. Consistently, and I mean consistently, act on these activities when you're confronted by cues and want to give in. Begin an incompatible activity as soon as you feel like overeating. In a remarkably short time, you'll begin to conquer the negative behavior that leads to overeating.

STEP TWO: OVERCOME YOUR IMPULSES AND URGES

If you're like most people trying to lose weight, you probably think that you must be disciplined and resolute twenty-four hours a day, seven days a week. This is a willpower-driven mind-set, however, that is doomed for failure. When your willpower runs out of steam, you invariably break your resolutions. In the aftermath, you develop a sense of guilt that only undermines your efforts and makes further weight-control indiscretions all the more likely. I'm sure you can relate to this way of thinking because it has been a part of your life for far too long.

Now here's something to sit still for: you do not have to be strong twenty-four hours a day, seven days a week.

Read that sentence again: you do not have to be strong twenty-four hours a day, seven days a week. The truth is, most of the fattening damage you do to yourself is inflicted at very isolated points in time. What this means is that your eating isn't eternally out of control; it's out of control only at certain times, during what I call *impulse moments*. These are brief periods of time, lasting no more than two or three minutes, in which you forget your resolve, you react without thinking, and you break your momentum by caving in to the urge to overeat or binge. Although they seem to come out of the blue, impulse moments are activated by cues in your environment, by your thoughts and feelings, by physical cravings for certain foods, and in response to certain events and circumstances.

You can expect to experience four to seven impulse moments during the day. An impulse moment can occur at specific times—for instance, at 5:30 P.M., when you get home from work, feeling like chewed twine after a long day. It can happen when you walk by a bakery and are enticed by the sight and smell of fresh pastries in the window. It can happen after a fight with your spouse, and suddenly you're stuffing your face with handfuls of M&M's. It can happen when, for no apparent reason, you start craving a certain food. It can happen any time, any place, in response to any event; just count on it because it will happen.

Impulse moments are critical for you to manage, because they have the unfortunate potential to derail even the best of efforts. When they hit, if you are not managing those impulses with a great degree of awareness and conscious resolve, then you are going to go spiraling back into your habitually self-destructive eating behavior every time. It's like getting to the finish line, only to have a trip wire stretched out in front of you—and boom, you're kissing the pavement.

That is why you need a real strategy worked out in advance with which to manage these impulse moments: otherwise you'll fall flat on your face. You need an advance plan for avoiding these moments, or at least outlasting them, one that takes into account the powerful negative pull of your past bad habits and programming, and the real-world challenges you face every day.

The best defense for heading off impulses, urges, and cravings is twofold. First, you must audit your day in order to figure when impulse moments are most likely to hit. That way, you're in a better position to avoid them by changing your routine, changing your schedule, or changing your environment.

Think about the following: what traps you into overeating? Is it a certain time of the day? Is it the people you hang out with? Is it paired with some type of activity, like watching TV? Do you get the urge to eat in certain places, like your car or your office? Do you turn to food when you're tired after work? So think about your impending day, where food is likely to be and what situations might trigger the impulse to eat. I want you to know where and when you could be hijacked by impulses, urges, and cravings, because they are to be expected.

The second part of your defense involves your response to impulse moments. What I want you to do is plan very carefully what you are going to do at those moments when you have the urge to binge or overeat. The very same activities you listed as part of your work above are activities you can purposely choose to engage in when these impulse moments strike. As soon as you feel the impulse, begin engaging, deliberately, in the incompatible substitute. Trust me, as soon as you do this, you will stop thinking about food and your desire to overeat will weaken. When you switch gears and start engaging in substitute activities, you change your train of thought, you change your routine, and you change your entire way of coping. Yes, this requires a little bit of energy, but the good news is that impulse moments pass as quickly as they hit—in an instant, poof, they're gone.

Many times, I've been sitting at my desk, engaged in a conference call that might drag on for hours. Before long, I'm feeling so hungry that I could eat the paint off the wall. Conference call over, I look at the clock. It's 6 o'clock and time for my tennis match. I start changing into my tennis clothes, I grab my gear, I race over to the courts. In the midst of this, all of a sudden I'm not hungry, I'm not even thinking about food, and I don't even consider grabbing something to eat along the way because I'm focused on my upcoming tennis match. I got through the moment. I did not give in to it. It passed—because my attention was diverted elsewhere.

However strong your own impulses, you should respond constructively so that you can overcome the tough stuff when it hits. Manage your impulse moments with a clear-cut plan, with a purpose, and you will bring much needed order into your life. Where before you might have surrendered to your impulses, now you will win and achieve what you want.

STEP THREE: CHANGE YOUR EATING STYLE

If you're overweight, then I know that you eat in a style that leads to overeating: eating too fast, eating while watching TV, eating far beyond the point of fullness, and so forth. When you eat like this, you shovel in an enormous number of calories in a very short period of time without even realizing it, and these calories are turned into body fat.

If you eat too fast, you won't feel full until it's too late. This is because after you begin a meal, it takes about twenty minutes for your body to send a message to your brain to switch off your appetite. But with rapid-fire eating, your brain does not get these "stop eating" signals until you have already stuffed yourself with too many calories. Whenever you eat too rapidly, you get hungry again more quickly than if you had eaten at a slower pace.

The encouraging news is that you can change these fattening habits with incompatible behaviors, too. For example, you can't wolf down a meal in split seconds if you take breaks during the meal. Taking breaks is incompatible with fast eating.

When Glenn, a former patient of mine, felt ready to shed the 50 pounds he needed to lose, he made only one change at first. A habitually fast eater, Glenn learned to put his utensils down after each bite. From counting his caloric intake at meals, we discovered that he had slashed his calories practically in half just by using this delaying tactic, yet he still felt satisfied even though he was eating much less. Glenn felt neither deprived nor threatened by this change; it was no big sacrifice. Each week, he would drop anywhere from 1 to 2 pounds, without much effort on his part.

As soon as this one simple change—slowing down his eating— became a matter of routine with Glenn, he knew he had the confidence and resolve to move on to other changes that ultimately brought him permanent weight loss. Making one small change at a time gave him the impetus to make other livable-for-life changes.

If you look at Table 4, you'll see that there are numerous incompatible behaviors you can employ to change your eating style. Please study this table carefully. Mastering even one or two of these changes will liberate you from counterproductive eating behavior and dramatically reduce your weight.

By employing these incompatible behaviors, you take the entire process of overeating off automatic pilot. If you're not already doing some of these things, start now. Otherwise you'll just become another

TABLE 4. INCOMPATIBLE BEHAVIORS TO SUBSTITUTE

TO CHANGE THIS EATING HABIT . . .	SUBSTITUTE THESE INCOMPATIBLE BEHAVIORS:
Fast eating	• After your food is placed in front of you, wait five minutes before you eat it. • Place small mouthfuls of food on your fork or in your spoon. • Completely swallow food from each mouthful before you add any more to your fork or spoon. • Put your utensils down between bites. • Use smaller utensils—a cocktail fork, for example—no soup spoons, ladles, or otherwise oversize tableware for shoveling in food. • Consciously take time to taste, chew, and savor the food you eat. • Stretch out your meals, making them last thirty minutes instead of five or ten, to allow for a reduction in hunger. One way to do this is to take a five-minute break about ten minutes into your meal. • Take sips of water or other noncaloric beverages between bites. • Introduce a one- or two-minute delay between courses.
Eating oversize portions	• Measure your food if you're afraid of overeating. • Use a smaller plate for your meals. • Purchase single-serving foods. • At restaurants, order one meal and ask for two plates so that you can split the meal with your spouse, date, or other dinner companion.

(continued on next page)

To change this eating habit . . .	Substitute these incompatible behaviors:
Eating oversize portions (continued)	• Avoid ordering super-size meals; opt for regular or kiddie portions instead.
Eating leftovers	• Put away all the food involved in preparing a meal. • Clear the table of serving plates. • Leave the table after you've finished eating. • Have someone else clean leftovers off the plates after meals. • Leave some food on your plate. • Purchase food in smaller packages or quantities so that you rarely have leftovers.
Eating while standing or on the move	• Localize your eating: select one area of your home—your dining room, breakfast nook, or some other area reserved only for eating—and eat *all* of your food at a designated table in that area. That includes regular meals, snacks, and beverages. • Never eat while driving in your car; standing in front of your open refrigerator; reading a book, magazine, or newspaper; sitting in your bed; or talking on the phone. In other words, do not pair other behaviors with eating. Doing so only distracts your attention from your eating behavior, and you will lose all sense and awareness of how much you are consuming.
Sampling food while cooking	• Place a small portion of the food on a plate; sit down and taste it. • Chew sugar-free gum while cooking. • Minimize your time in the kitchen.
Eating in several rooms in your home	• Designate only one place—your kitchen or dining room table—and eat all your meals there.
Nighttime eating	• Brush your teeth in the evening to signal that you've finished eating for the night.
Snacking while watching television	• Eat only in your designated eating place—at your kitchen or dining room table. • Eliminate all distractions while eating—including television (turn it off).
Overeating at parties or social events	• Eat low-calorie foods before you go. • Concentrate on people and conversation, not on food. • Position yourself away from the food or buffet table.

casualty of unsuccessful behavior. So behave differently when it comes to food, resolving to push food out of the center of your life. If you continue to eat the way you've always eaten, you will continue to stay the way you always have been. But when you begin to do different things, you'll begin to stimulate additional changes. Organize yourself and your day in a way that moves you up the success ladder. Believe me, when you do these things, your weight will start peeling off, and your life will become so much more ordered and productive. You'll begin to enjoy a whole new way of eating and living, one that is so much more satisfying that you will not want to ever turn back.

New Payoffs from New Behaviors

At this point, we need to revisit the issue of payoffs. Most of the activities you and I have listed and talked about in this chapter will generate the very same payoffs that you used to get from food and from overeating. Take exercise, for example. Exercising, whether it involves going for a jog or working in your garden, produces surges in feel-good brain chemicals, just as overeating does, but without the disastrous consequences. Relaxation, meditation, listening to music: all of these generate the payoffs of physiological calm or emotional relief. Even volunteering—helping others by giving your time and talents—has been shown in research to produce a sense of calm, well-being, and other incredibly positive physiological changes in mental and physical health. Obligatory activities like doing housework or cleaning out your closets can give you a sense of accomplishment, while taking your mind off food and weakening your desire to overeat. Using the incompatible behaviors listed in the table above, you can eat less food, enjoy it more, and still feel satisfied while effortlessly losing weight in the process.

Choosing new behaviors, ones that are constructive and positive, will seep into other areas of your life, improving the way you may now be living. Take your emotional responses, for example. If your life is characterized by boredom, depression, or any of a number of similar traits, you can minimize these or eliminate them, and the reactive eating that they trigger, with new behaviors. It has long been my contention that bored people are boring, and that depressed people are depressing. If bored people would do more interesting things—that is, not act so boring—they would have a very different experience of life. If depressed people—even those who are biochemically depressed—would "act" more enthusiastic about life, then they'd be happier. The adage that "You can't get anywhere unless you start" is definitely true. You can't get happier if you do not get into the game. By getting into the game, by behaving the way you want your life to be, you give yourself the chance to experience the payoffs that come from those kinds of behaviors. Create what you want by doing what you can.

I could go on and on. I just want you to see that, as things go, just about every constructive activity you can substitute for overeating can become a positive force in your life and will generate payoffs that are healthy and emotionally uplifting. Whenever you choose a health-enhancing or life-enriching activity and perform it on a regular basis, that activity becomes a habit itself—a positive addiction, if you will. With this comes not only better looks and health, but also a richer, more satisfying life.

When you continue to choose healthier behaviors and disconnect from toxic, short-term payoffs, you'll discover that there is another payoff system at work: the positive payoffs that come from the newfound mastery in your life. To illustrate what I mean, let me tell you what I wish you to think, say, and feel once you become the captain of your own behavior again and you achieve your goals:

> It feels good to be in control. When I get up in the morning, I'm excited about the day. No longer ashamed of my reflection in the mirror, I like what I see and I'm proud of who I am. I've found the discipline to eat according to my needs rather than be driven by self-destructive habits, impulses, or diets. Able to face the day without overeating, I no longer allow habit and cues to dictate my life. I have a rock-solid foundation for my new eating habits that cannot be destroyed. I live more fully now that my body is functioning better, and I am free to forget about food and get on with living. Gone are my old excesses, and I now have time to use for productive, enjoyable activities. Whether learning a new sport, reading a book, or writing a poem, I enjoy it more be-

cause I am not overeating. I've discovered skills I didn't think I had. I have the confidence to get involved in new pursuits, take a course, or change my profession. When I walk into a room, people are cheering for me because they have known and shared my struggle. I'm asked what I've done to look so great. I finally feel good in my clothes—no more pants that won't fasten across my stomach and no more outfits intended to hide my fatness. As my body gets thinner, healthier, and more athletic, I experience it with greater awareness and pleasure. I have gained new satisfaction and self-respect in whatever I choose to do. I know life won't be a bed of roses in the future any more than it is today, but I know how to deal with difficulties. I know how to handle life with greater maturity. I know how to cope with life in positive ways without escaping into food. I am no longer going in circles, but moving forward with tremendous clarity about why I am in this world and what I am supposed to do while I am here. There is adventure in my day and joy in my heart. I have learned to live a life of meaning and significance.

I just offer these words to get you percolating and thinking about the payoffs you'll experience from healthy behavior, and about the way you want your life to be. Go back and reread this passage, daily if you wish, using it as a positive affirmation and to keep familiarizing yourself with the essence of this program and why you are doing it for yourself. When you use every key and go through every door in this program, you will feel like nothing can stop you on your journey to actually living these words.

By "behaving your way to success," you will begin to lose even more weight. Once you begin to behave differently, in ways that reflect your weight-management priorities, then you will begin to enjoy the rewards and benefits that flow from those kinds of behaviors. I can tell you that as a good barometer, if people in your life do not find it glaringly obvious that you have changed the way you live, act, think, and feel, then you have not made dramatic enough changes. You make a difference when you do different. When you behave like a winner, you are a winner.

8

Key Five:
High-Response Cost,
High-Yield Nutrition

Unlock the Door to Food Control

> *I never worry about diets. The only carrots that*
> *interest me are the number you get in a diamond.*
> —MAE WEST

KEY #5: HIGH-RESPONSE COST,
HIGH-YIELD NUTRITION.

Be aware that certain foods lead to a considerable amount of mindless, uncontrollable overeating. If you eliminate or cut back on these
foods, you will control your weight automatically, and live in peace
with food.

If you are eating without any degree of control, stuffing your face
with everything that doesn't move, then you need more than anything else what I call a *behavioral approach* to food and nutrition. This
is a way to eat that tames your hunger, stops destructive patterns of
eating, and enables you to regain control over food and how much
you eat. It is designed to build on what you already know about food
and good nutrition, so that you do not have to start from scratch. I
call it my High-Response Cost, High-Yield Food Plan, which means
that it focuses on choosing foods that produce and reinforce lasting
weight loss and control. As we go through this chapter together, you
will see why this plan works so powerfully to help you lose weight, ef-
fectively and permanently, without turning your life upside down or
driving you nuts.

This approach runs absolutely counter to what most "diets" push, which is a metabolic approach to weight loss, usually employing puritanical restrictions of certain food groups or special combinations of food that promise miraculous fat burning. These approaches may work for a short time, but as soon as you return to your old ways of eating, your weight returns, with interest. This key—high-response cost, high-yield nutrition—unlocks the door to food control so that you are no longer a prisoner of binges, cravings, and fixations on food. You will discover some truths about food that I'm sure no one has ever told you before, and you will rely on important food realities to achieve and maintain a healthy weight, instead of resorting to another bizarre fad diet or gimmicky program that will keep you from ever attaining permanent weight loss.

SUE ANN'S STORY

Since I believe it's always helpful to have a model or example to illustrate key concepts, allow me to share with you a brief story of a former patient of mine, Sue Ann, who was enrolled in my program for chronically overweight patients. She was twenty-four and a single mother of a young son when she entered the program, and had already eaten her way up to 250 pounds. Her eating was way out of control, characterized by one binge after another. She lived to eat, and hated herself every minute for it.

Sue Ann's husband had abandoned his family several years before. Jobless most of the time, he had been unable to support them, and so Sue Ann was forced to do the juggling act of mother and breadwinner. She was holding down not one but two jobs, working for a maid service by day and as a cashier by night. Her means barely covered the minimum. The ferocious demands on her time, coupled with the mind-numbing fatigue of her long days, wedged her into a habitual pattern of buying and bingeing on fast foods, or any food that was convenient and required little or no preparation. Sue Ann never took the time to do any cooking or food preparation, simply because she was too busy and too tired after working all day to worry about eating right. It was easier to grab and go, picking up fast food, carryout, and other unhealthy junk food. This had been her routine for years, and now she was living the consequences. Food had become not only her time-saver, but also her companion and consoler. Many times, she would buy a whole chocolate cake for herself when she felt tired and sorry for herself, and cry as she consumed it piece by piece.

By the time she entered my program, Sue Ann's health had begun to deteriorate, while her weight continued to climb. She had high blood pressure, dangerously high cholesterol, and had been diagnosed as a borderline diabetic. Clearly, we had challenges ahead of us.

For Sue Ann to get well, to stop her self-sabotage, and to ultimately stabilize her weight at a healthy level, we had to first work on a new life strategy for her. Her lifestyle was chaotic, out of control, and it was clearly supporting and sustaining what she had become. The scales of her life were tipped too much in favor of self-defeating behavior, and as a result, she was living a distinctly unbalanced lifestyle, and this was contributing in a big way to her weight problem.

Sue Ann had to dump that lifestyle, with all the wrong things that had been working to the disadvantage of her weight and health, and start living anew. This required on her part a commitment to quit one of her jobs, move in with a relative until she could get on her feet financially, and basically reevaluate her priorities and options. In short, she had to recreate her own experience.

Once Sue Ann had begun to deconstruct her world and put it back together again—with fewer time constraints and pressures—she was ready to work on her weight, food choices, and behavior.

Her work focused on the foods she was eating. The fast food, the easy-to-fix foods, and all the grab-and-go stuff she was choosing were doing nothing more than promoting rapid, uncontrollable, mindless eating, and the result of this behavior was an ever-increasing weight gain. Sue Ann's problem with food was mostly behavioral, and it had to be solved behaviorally.

What we settled upon was the following: Sue Ann agreed to eat foods from a list that I would give her. It wasn't a diet, just a list of foods. What's more, I told her that if she still wanted junk food and fast food after eating foods from the list, she could do so. That was it. That was the extent of the plan.

When Sue Ann came to see me following a week of eating from

the list, I asked her, "How did it go? Were you able to eat from the list?"

Her face lit up. She told me in amazement, "I did it. It wasn't as hard as I thought it would be. I just ate from the list. As for junk food, usually I felt fine going without it. I lost eight pounds, and I feel different."

So each week thereafter, Sue Ann renewed our agreement to eat from my food list, and while not every week was perfect, she began to feel in better control of food and more confident that she could change her eating behavior. After a few months, she was buying smaller clothes, zipping up jeans that hadn't fit in years, and feeling so much better about herself that she wanted to keep going.

The upshot of this story is that it took Sue Ann ten months to get to her goal weight of 120 pounds. A huge factor in her transformation was, of course, rebalancing her life so that she could take care of her health, and spend more quality time pursuing things that would be life-enriching and not revolve so much around food.

As her life began to change, she began to feel more energized, physically and emotionally. Her desire to binge on emotion lost its grip on her life. She gradually took up a walking program, and that made losing weight so much easier. Sometimes easy-to-eat foods like fast food and pizza were her weak points. But she didn't eliminate them from her life altogether. She just limited them to occasional indulgences.

In losing all that weight, she had lost one half of herself, and in the process gained so much more. Sue Ann learned what it meant to make choices for the health of her body, reversing the health complications of obesity through good nutrition, so that she could regain the strength and energy she needed to get on with her life.

Maybe you can relate to Sue Ann's experience. Maybe this is where you are right now. If so, you need a new approach to food, something doable but not drastic that you can do, starting today, to regain control over food. This is exactly what we will do in this key.

Let's begin by taking a nutritional assessment to examine more closely your food choices, and whether they are working for you or against you.

NUTRITIONAL ASSESSMENT

Most people misjudge how poorly they really eat or how often they consume various foods, and as a result, have no idea of how their food choices are driving weight-gaining behavior. By completing this assessment, you'll take a big step toward understanding where you are nutritionally, and where you could be. You'll confront the ways in which you're harming your health and stonewalling your weight-control efforts. Keep these questions—and your answers—in mind as you continue to work through the rest of this key.

This is a multiple-choice assessment organized into seven separate sections. For each section, answer the questions honestly, then total up your score at the end of the section. The points you receive for each answer appear at the right. After completing the assessment, you'll have a total of seven different scores. How to interpret those scores is discussed at the end of the assessment.

Section 1: MEAL & SNACKS

1. How many meals do you eat each day?
   a. 3 meals and 2 snacks — 3
   b. 3 meals and 1 snack — 2
   c. 2 meals — 1
   d. 1 meal — 0

2. How often do you eat breakfast?
   a. Every day — 3
   b. 4 to 6 days a week — 2
   c. 1 to 3 days a week — 1
   d. Never — 0

3. Breakfast usually includes:
   a. An egg, whole-wheat toast or cereal, and fruit or fruit juice — 3
   b. A bowl of sugary cereal with milk, or pancakes with syrup — 2
   c. A doughnut — 1
   d. Nothing — 0

4. How would you characterize most of your dinners?
   a. Homecooked, with meat, chicken, or fish,   3
   vegetables, a salad
   b. Whatever I can pop into the microwave   2
   c. Eaten at a restaurant   1
   d. Eaten at a fast-food restaurant or as take out   0

5. How often do you eat at fast-food restaurants?
   a. Rarely   3
   b. 1 to 3 times a week   2
   c. 4 to 7 times a week   1
   d. More than 8 times a week   0

6. How often do you vary the foods you eat through the week?
   a. Very often   3
   b. Often   2
   c. Rarely   1
   d. Never—I eat the same foods all the time   0

7. How would you describe your snacking habits?
   a. I snack nutritiously, to supplement my diet with   3
   extra nutrients
   b. I occasionally snack   2
   c. I always seem to be snacking   1
   d. Snacking leads to a full-blown binge   0

8. For snacks, your typical choices are:
   a. Fresh fruits or vegetables, or nutritional drinks or   3
   bars
   b. Grain-based foods like pretzels, rice cakes,   2
   or crackers
   c. Chips like potato chips or taco chips, or other   1
   salty snack food
   d. Candy, cookies, or any type of sweet   0

YOUR SCORE FOR SECTION 1:

Section 2: NUTRIENT BALANCE

1. How many servings do you eat each day of grain products? (One serving = 1 slice of bread; or ½ cup cooked grain, such as pasta, rice or barley; or ½ cup of dry cereal. Do not include biscuits, croissants, cookies, cakes, or other high-fat/high-sugar choices)
   a. 3 or more servings a day   3
   b. 2 servings a day   2
   c. 1 serving a day   1
   d. None   0

2. How many servings of calcium-rich milk and dairy foods (like low-fat milk, low-fat yogurt, or reduced-fat cheese) do you eat each day? (One serving = 1 cup milk or yogurt, 1 ounce cheese, ½ cup canned salmon, or 4 ounces of tofu)
   a. 3   3
   b. 2   2
   c. 1   1
   d. None   0

3. How many servings do you eat each day of dark green leafy vegetables such as romaine lettuce, spinach, kale, or collard greens? (One serving = 1 cup raw or ½ cup cooked)
   a. 2 or more a day   3
   b. 1   2
   c. ½   1
   d. None   0

4. During the week, how many servings of orange or yellow vegetables or fruit do you eat? (Examples include winter squash, pumpkin, carrots, melons, peaches, and apricots. One serving = 1 cup raw, or ½ cup cooked)
   a. 3 or more   3
   b. 2   2
   c. 1   1
   d. None   0

5. During the week, how many servings do you eat of high vitamin C fruits? (Examples include citrus fruits, strawberries, or kiwi fruit. One serving = 1 piece of fruit, ½ cup juice, 1 cup of raw diced fruit)

   a. 3 or more   3
   b. 2   2
   c. 1   1
   d. None   0

6. During the week, how many servings of other vegetables do you eat? (Examples include broccoli, cauliflower, cabbage, brussels sprouts, summer squash, zucchini, green beans, turnips, or beets. One serving = ½ cup cooked or 1 cup raw)

   a. 5 or more   3
   b. 3 to 4   2
   c. 1 to 2   1
   d. None   0

7. During the week, do you eat at least one serving of lean red meat, or at least two servings of chicken or turkey?

   a. Yes   3
   b. Sometimes   2
   c. Never   1

YOUR SCORE FOR SECTION 2:

Section 3: FIBER

1. Are you generally aware of the fiber content in the foods you eat?

   a. Yes   3
   b. No   1

2. What type of cereal do you normally eat?

   a. Something high in fiber, usually with bran,   3
      or cooked oat bran
   b. A cooked cereal like oatmeal or cream of wheat   2
   c. A packaged cereal, one that's sweet   −2
   d. I never eat cereals of any kind   −3

3. What type of bread (including rolls, bagels, and muffins) do you usually eat?

    a. Whole-wheat, whole grain, or mixed grain   3

    b. Partial whole-wheat   2

    c. White bread   0

4. How often do you eat beans or legumes such as kidney beans, black beans, pinto beans, garbanzos, soybeans, lentils, or split peas?

    a. 5 or more times a week   3

    b. 2 to 4 times a week   2

    c. Once a week   1

    d. Never   0

5. How often do you eat cooked whole grains, such as brown rice, bulgur wheat, or barley?

    a. 5 or more times a week   3

    b. 2 to 4 times a week   2

    c. Once a week   1

    d. Never   0

6. How many servings of fresh or raw vegetables do you eat each day?

    a. 7 to 8 servings or more a day   3

    b. 4 to 6 servings a day   2

    c. 1 to 3 servings a day   1

    d. Hardly ever   0

YOUR SCORE FOR SECTION 3:

Section 4: SUGAR & PROCESSED CARBOHYDRATES

1. How often do you eat candy or cookies?

    a. Never, or a few times a year   3

    b. Several times a month   2

    c. A few times a week   −2

    d. Almost daily   −3

2. How often do you eat desserts (pies, cakes, or other baked sweets), other than fruit?

a.	Never, or a few times a year	3
b.	Several times a month	2
c.	A few times a week	−2
d.	Almost daily	−3

3. How often do you eat full-fat ice cream, milk shakes, or frozen desserts?

a.	Never, or a few times a year	3
b.	Several times a month	2
c.	A few times a week	−2
d.	Almost daily	−3

4. How often do you drink sugared sodas?

a.	Never, or a few times a year	3
b.	Several times a month	2
c.	A few times a week	−2
d.	Almost daily	−3

5. How often do you drink flavored coffees and similar beverages?

a.	Never, or a few times a year	3
b.	Several times a month	2
c.	A few times a week	−2
d.	Almost daily	−3

YOUR SCORE FOR SECTION 4:

Section 5: FAT INTAKE

1. When you eat bread, toast, bagels, or rolls, what type of spread do you put on them?

a.	Sugar-free fruit spreads, nonfat cream cheese, or nothing	3
b.	Jam	2
c.	Butter	1
d.	Margarine or cream cheese	0

2. How many times during a typical week do you eat processed meats, such as bacon, luncheon meats, sausage, hot dogs, or salami?
   a. Never   3
   b. 1 to 2 times a week   2
   c. 3 to 5 times a week   1
   d. Nearly every day   0

3. When you eat at a fast-food restaurant, do you usually order:
   a. A salad or other light entrée   3
   b. Hamburgers, but in junior or small-size servings   2
   c. Cheeseburger, hamburger, or other sandwich   1
   d. Any large-size sandwich, with fries   0

4. What do you ordinarily put on your salad?
   a. Nothing, or vinegar or lemon juice   3
   b. Reduced calorie or nonfat salad dressing   2
   c. Regular salad dressing or oil and vinegar   1
   d. Creamy salad dressings—the more, the better   0

5. How often do you eat red meat during a typical week?
   a. Once, or seldom   3
   b. 2 to 3 times a week   2
   c. 4 to 6 times a week   −2
   d. 7 or more times a week   −3

6. Which types of foods do you usually eat from the following two lists?

   High Saturated Fat Foods: red meat, hot dogs, sausage, bacon, luncheon meats, sour cream, butter, full-fat cheeses (cheddar, jack, Swiss, Brie, etc.), whole milk, 2% milk, cream, half-and-half, full-fat ice cream, and fried foods

   Low Saturated Fat Foods: poultry with skin removed, fish, low-fat dairy products (nonfat, skim, or 1% milk) vegetables, pasta, and legumes

   a. I eat mostly foods that are low in saturated fat   3
   b. I eat about the same from each list   1
   c. I eat mostly foods that are high in saturated fat   −3

7. When cooking with fats or oils, do you typically:
   a. Reduce the amount of fat in recipes, or substitute applesauce for fat ⟶ 3
   b. Use reduced-fat products, or oils high in monounsaturated fats (olive, canola) ⟶ 2
   c. Use other vegetable oils (soy, safflower, corn) ⟶ 1
   d. Use margarine, butter, or vegetable shortening ⟶ 0

YOUR SCORE FOR SECTION 5:

Section 6: SALT

1. How often do you salt your foods when cooking or eating?
   a. Never or rarely ⟶ 3
   b. Occasionally ⟶ 2
   c. Usually ⟶ 1
   d. Always ⟶ 0

2. How often do you eat salted chips or nuts, luncheon meats, or crackers?
   a. Never or rarely ⟶ 3
   b. A few times a week ⟶ 2
   c. Once a day ⟶ 1
   d. Several times a day ⟶ 0

3. To season your foods, you typically use:
   a. Herbs, lemon juice, or other non-sodium spices ⟶ 3
   b. A salt substitute ⟶ 2
   c. Soy sauce or teriyaki sauce ⟶ 1
   d. Salt ⟶ 0

YOUR SCORE FOR SECTION 6:

Section 7: FLUIDS

1. How much water do you drink each day?
   a. 8 to 10 cups ⟶ 3
   b. 5 to 7 cups ⟶ 2

c.	3 to 4 cups	1
d.	Less than 3 cups	0

2. How many servings of caffeine-containing beverages do you drink each day? (One serving = 1 cup of coffee, 2 cups of tea, or 12 ounces of a soft drink)

a.	One or none	3
b.	2	2
c.	3 to 4	1
d.	More than 4	0

YOUR SCORE FOR SECTION 7:

INTERPRETING YOUR SCORES

Let's look at your scores for each separate section so that you will have a clear idea of how you're doing in specific areas of your nutrition.

Section 1: If you scored above 16 points, you have developed some excellent meal and snack habits. Eating three meals a day, with healthy snacks in between, is important to weight control since it keeps your metabolism humming along throughout the day. Equally important to weight control is breakfast; studies have found that breakfast eaters have fewer cravings and hunger pangs later in the day, and are better able to control their appetites at other meals. This section also underlines the importance of eating a variety of foods, including healthy snacks, so that your body is fueled with the broadest range of nutrients possible. A score under 16 indicates the need for improvement in these areas.

Section 2: If you scored more than 14 points, your present diet is abundant in vitamin and minerals. Grains supply B vitamins. Dairy products provide calcium, which is important not only for bone building but also for regulating body weight. Green vegetables are vital sources of folic acid, a vitamin now known to protect against a range of diseases, including heart disease and cancer. You get vitamin A and other protective nutrients from orange and yellow vegetables, and vitamin C from citrus fruits. If your score shows you're skimping in any of these areas, it's time for a nutritional overhaul.

Section 3: If your score is 12 or higher, you're well on the road to high-fiber eating. That's good, because fiber provides a number of weight- and appetite-controlling advantages (not to mention excellent digestive health). If you flunked the fiber part of this assessment, begin eating more whole grains, beans and legumes—and start reading labels to ascertain the fiber content of foods. You need between 20 and 35 grams of fiber daily.

Section 4: If you scored 10 or higher (preferably closer to 15), congratulations. You've successfully shunned a class of foods—sugar and processed foods—that in long-term excess burdens your metabolism. Eating too much sugar makes you hungry for more sugar, and so a vicious cycle ensues. The overabundance of sugar, sugary processed foods, along with saturated fats from animal sources, shoulders much of the blame for "insulin resistance," a condition that occurs when the body builds up a tolerance to the hormone insulin. Insulin's job is to keep your blood sugar within normal ranges—neither too high nor too low—by shuttling that blood sugar into your muscle cells for energy. With insulin resistance, your body is less efficient at controlling blood sugar, which piles up in your bloodstream, creating a toxic metabolic environment. Many experts believe that insulin resistance encourages obesity and leads to diabetes and heart disease.

Section 5: If your score is above 13, you do a good job of curbing the fat in your diet. A low score, or one that's in negative territory, should be a loud wake-up call. Reevaluate what you're doing. Eating the wrong types of fat, namely the saturated variety, can harm your health and make you so much more susceptible to life-shortening illnesses.

Section 6: If your score is over 6, your intake of sodium (the mineral in salt) is well controlled. But if your score is less than 6, start reducing your sodium by controlling the salt shaker. Salty foods also tend to be high in fat—a combination that is addictive in its taste appeal and compels you to devour greasy foods like potato chips in ever-increasing amounts. But when it comes to salt, less is better. Cutting back on salt can reduce high blood pressure in people who are sensitive to sodium's effects.

Section 7: If your score is above 4, you're watering your body well and monitoring your intake of caffeine. Both are good habits for people who want to stay healthy. Water is required by every cell in your body for peak health.

• • •

Take some time to go back and read through your answers. You've identified the nutritional choices you're making—choices that either harm you or help you. Do yourself the honor of treating this time of reflection seriously. Your work here in assessing your nutritional choices is an important move toward changing them, and you will want to be very aware of those choices, from this point forward, so that you can do the necessary work required to achieve control over food.

FOOD CONTROL: HIGH-RESPONSE COST FOOD VERSUS LOW-RESPONSE COST FOOD

For you to achieve food control, I want to stress something very important from the outset: food has a *behavioral effect*. Certain foods keep bad eating habits alive. Take fast foods. Most can be polished off in no time flat, before your satiety or satisfaction signals kick in. Before you realize it, you've eaten much more food than you need, and considerably more than you wanted. Foods like these promote a counterproductive behavior pattern that you're trying to stop: fast, mindless, and uncontrolled overeating. So if you are going to manage your weight with any degree of control, you have to recognize which foods work against you in a behavioral sense, so you can avoid or limit them as much as possible, and which foods work for you.

To bring this behavioral aspect of food into sharper focus, it helps to think of your food choices as either:

High-response cost foods, or

Low-response cost foods

What exactly do I mean by "high-response cost foods" and "low-response cost foods?" Let's explore this in depth—what it means to you in terms of achieving greater behavioral control over your eating and your ability to lose pounds.

HIGH-RESPONSE COST FOODS

High-response cost foods are those that require a great deal of work and effort to prepare and to eat. The work output required to ingest these foods is high, whereas the calorie payoff is low—and healthy.

A good example of a high-response cost food is raw broccoli. It is coarse and takes a lot of chewing and grinding to get it down. Another is a sunflower seed still in its hull. You've got to work a whole lot at extracting a little bit of meat from that tiny seed. You can't just knock back a handful, either; you've got to exert yourself for every bite. Foods like beef or chicken are high-response cost foods, too. Usually, you have to take them out of your freezer, defrost them, and cook them before they're edible. You wouldn't just grab some raw meat and start eating.

Another example of a high-response cost food—and one that is probably in your pantry right now—is soup. Behavioral scientists have studied soup as a weight-control tool for decades, discovering in numerous experiments that it reduces hunger and controls caloric intake. Why is this so? Because soup generally takes a long time to eat, prolonging mealtime and thereby allowing the body's natural hunger signals to kick in. What's more, soup is filling, so that by the time you've finished your soup course, you are less likely to want much else. One study I read found that a group of volunteers effortlessly lost eight pounds in ten weeks, doing nothing out of the ordinary except eating a bowl of soup prior to lunch or dinner! (If you try this technique, let me suggest that you eat lighter, broth-based soups such as vegetable soups because they are less fattening than thick, cream-laden soups.)

Fresh fruits and vegetables, beans and legumes, meats, poultry, fish, whole grains, and certain cereals are all examples of other high-response cost foods. You will find an extensive list of these foods in Appendix B, and you should refer to this list for meal planning.

To sum up, high-response cost foods:

- Take considerable time and effort to fix

- Require a great deal of chewing and ingestion energy

- Cannot be eaten quickly

- Are not "convenience foods" in any sense of the word.

The fact that you must take time to prepare these foods, and that they take effort to chew and eat is a real advantage to weight control. Why? *Because high-response cost foods defeat impulse eating and therefore support control.* Mealtime behavior becomes so much more manageable when you choose mostly high-response cost foods.

LOW-RESPONSE COST FOODS

By contrast, low-response cost foods are easily ingested, overly convenient, and require little or no preparation. An excellent example of a low-response cost food is a sour cream–and–bean burrito from a fast-food Mexican restaurant. When you eat one, you don't even have to chomp on the burrito; it just slithers down your throat in a few quick gulps. What happens is that you consume an incredibly high number of calories and fat in a very short period of time.

Your body's natural stop-eating signals don't even have time to activate when you eat low-response cost foods. Remember, it takes about 20 minutes from the time you eat something until the hypothalamus in your brain turns off your appetite. There's absolutely no way that burrito can offer any satisfying effects when it's overly easy to wolf it down in a matter of seconds. So you keep eating more and more of this stuff until you've eaten way beyond the point of fullness; and the unfortunate fact is that you're overfed with unnecessary calories and fat.

Other examples of low-response cost foods are candy, chocolate, puddings, any high-calorie convenience food, foods you grab and eat on the run, foods eaten directly from their storage containers, easy-to-prepare processed foods, and any food classified as "junk food." Among the most notorious low-response cost foods are fast foods, such as hamburgers, cheeseburgers, fried chicken sandwiches, fish sandwiches, hot dogs, croissant sandwiches, breakfast muffins or biscuits, burritos, tacos, fried chicken, chicken nuggets, french fries, and milk shakes. Snack foods such as potato chips, taco chips, corn chips, pretzels, cheese curls, and butter- or oil-popped popcorn are low-response cost foods. So are cookies, brownies, cakes, snack cakes, pies, and other baked goods. For a complete list of low-response cost foods, refer to Appendix B.

Low-response cost foods bully you into fast, uncontrolled eating, and this type of mindless eating is a behavior you must try to eliminate, since it figures so significantly in obesity. Trying to change unwanted behavior, even under the best of circumstances, is difficult enough. You certainly don't want to add to the difficulty by eating foods that invite the very behavior you want to eliminate! We eat too fast anyway, but our choice of foods—easy-to-ingest, low-response cost foods—makes that behavior worse.

But there are other consequences, too. If a low-response cost food is crispy with sharp edges—such as taco or tortilla chips—you can literally lacerate your throat. I'm not kidding! According to one study I read, the chief cause of throat tears in this country is eating taco chips too fast, without chewing them. It's like swallowing a buzz saw. There's more: the number one mouth wound seen by doctors is burn, caused by gulping down hot food too fast.

To sum up, low-response cost foods:

- Are overly convenient and easily accessible—foods that are easy to grab and eat in no time flat

- Invite and promote fast, uncontrolled eating

- Need little or no preparation time

- Require little chewing or effort to eat. The food slides down your throat, and you barely have to chew it

- Melt in your mouth

- Can be eaten too easily straight from a package or container

Low-response cost foods lead to uncontrolled eating because they tend to be soft, ingested too easily, and overly convenient. In short, they have a negative effect on your eating behavior. Suffice it to say, you should avoid eating low-response cost foods, or at least limit them to the rare splurge.

UNDERSTANDING THE NUTRITIONAL YIELD OF FOOD

If you are ever to get your weight under control and experience true weight loss freedom, you must understand that food has *nutritional yield*. This term describes whether a particular food is a good source of nutrients, without being too high in calories. Some foods have a high yield; some have a low yield.

HIGH-YIELD FOODS

High-yield foods are those that supply a lot of nutrients—in the form of carbohydrate, protein, fat, vitamins, minerals, fiber, and other food components—relative to the amount of calories they contain. Take carrots, for example. One carrot delivers virtually all the health-promoting beta-carotene you need in a day, and is extremely low in calories (about 30 calories per carrot). You're getting lots of nutrition for very few calories. When you're on a limited budget of calories, you naturally want to get the best nutritional buy for your buck. High-yield foods give you that kind of nutritional bargain.

High-yield foods are generally those of a more pure, basic variety, and are closer to the state in which they are found in nature. They have not been substantially changed during food processing, and thus are not usually laced with added sugar, fat, additives, and other health-defeating ingredients.

High-yield foods such as fruits and vegetables are colorful too, a sign that they are plentiful in important food factors that reduce your risk of disease. To be the beneficiary of this healing power, you should eat by color. Fruits and vegetables that are red or purple, such as blueberries, red cabbage, tomatoes, or red peppers, are endowed with important food factors that reduce your risk of diseases. Apricots, carrots, and sweet potatoes—all orange foods—are loaded with beta-carotene. Yellow and green fruits and vegetables contain important natural chemicals that protect your body in numerous ways. What's more, high-yield grains, as well as fruits and vegetables, are loaded with fiber, a beneficial constituent that naturally makes you feel full.

Not coincidentally, most high-yield foods also happen to be

high-response cost foods. Returning to our example of raw broccoli, the high-response cost food I mentioned above, this vegetable has a substantial nutritional yield, providing a treasure trove of vitamins, mineral, fiber, and plant chemicals, which are constituents of plant foods that have disease-fighting biological activity. Raw broccoli is thus an example of a high-response cost, high-yield food.

Low-Yield Foods

Many of the food choices we make are low-yield. These are foods that provide an excess of calories, in relation to the nutrients they contain. They impart very little, if any, nutritional value in the way of vitamins, minerals, fiber, and other beneficial constituents. Put another way, they have a load of calories packed into a very small amount of real food. Sugar and fats are examples of low-yield foods. They are very high in calories but practically devoid of nutrition, and for these reasons, they are best kept off-limits if you want to successfully control your weight.

Keep in mind, too, that low-yield foods are engineered to be addictive—loaded with sugar, extra fat, calories, too much salt, and unhealthy additives—and of questionable nutritional value. What's more, they are processed and refined; that is, they have been milled or altered in some fashion that devalues their nutrition by extracting fiber and other nutrients.

You can often tell a low-yield food by its color, too. If a fruit or vegetable that is naturally colorful looks as faded as a motel tan, then it's a sure bet that its nutrients have faded with it.

It's not surprising to point out that low-yield foods are mostly low-response cost foods—all weak in their nutritional value and saddled with unwanted and entirely unnecessary junk. These foods challenge your body and work at cross-purposes to weight loss, behavioral control, and good health.

In the table below is a brief list of high-yield and low-yield foods. You'll find an expanded list of these foods in Appendix B.

TABLE 5. COMPARATIVE LIST OF HIGH- AND LOW-YIELD FOODS

High-Yield Foods	Low-Yield Foods
Whole Grains, Breads, and Rice	
• Whole grains (wheat, oats, barley, millet) • Whole grain breads, rolls, bagels, crackers, and muffins • Whole grain and high-fiber cereals • Whole grain pastas • Brown rice	• Croissants • Fried rice • Doughnuts and pastries • Sweet rolls • Cookies
Vegetables	
• Beans sprouts, broccoli, Brussels sprouts, cabbage, carrots, cauliflower, corn, cucumbers, green beans, leafy vegetables, legumes, mushrooms, potatoes, summer and winter squash, tomatoes, sweet potatoes, yams	• French-fried potatoes, fried vegetables • Vegetables packaged in sauce
Fruits	
• All fresh fruits, especially apples, apricots, bananas, berries, cantaloupe, citrus fruits, peaches, pears • Natural fruit juices • Canned or frozen fruits, unsweetened or packed in water or juice	• Canned or frozen fruits, sweetened or packed in syrup • Fruit rolls • Fruit drinks
Proteins and Protein Substitutes	
• Eggs and egg whites, fish, lean meats, legumes, tempeh, tofu	• Hot dogs, luncheon meats, nuts, sausage bacon, fried fish, fried poultry

Dairy Products	
• Nonfat, skim, and 1% milk • Nonfat products such as buttermilk, cottage cheese, and yogurt • Soy milk (fortified) • Nonfat ice milks and sherbets	• Whole milk • Whole milk products such as cheese, cottage cheese, custard, milk shakes, pudding, and ice cream
Beverages	
• Water • Herbal teas	• Sugared soft drinks • Alcoholic beverages

HUNGER SUPPRESSORS AND HUNGER DRIVERS

Before moving forward, there is one more issue to address with regard to high-response cost, high-yield nutrition, and that's how to get more satisfaction from less food so that you won't overeat or be so ruled by cravings and urges.

High-response cost, high-yield foods are *hunger suppressors*, meaning they can control and curb your hunger. Because they take longer to eat, your body has more time to receive stop-eating signals from your hypothalamus. By the time you chew and swallow these foods, you're starting to feel full, so there is little chance that you will overeat. You will be amazed at how little food you'll eat, yet how full and satisfied you'll feel after eating it.

Also, high-response cost, high-yield foods are often abundant in fiber, a weight-control ally that promotes feelings of fullness, stabilizes your blood sugar, and thus keeps your hunger at bay so that you're less likely to overeat.

Where hunger is concerned, low-response cost, low-yield foods are a different story altogether. We've already seen that these foods stimulate fast eating with no corresponding effect on fullness—all of which goes to show that low-response cost, low-yield foods are *hunger drivers*.

There's more: any food that is overly processed with sugar and refined carbohydrates, as many low-response cost, low-yield foods are, will create a seesaw effect in your blood sugar, driving it up, then letting it nose-dive. Low blood sugar leads to hunger and cravings. When you eat low-response cost, low-yield foods, your hunger mechanisms become totally ungovernable.

So you see: low-response cost, low-yield foods not only encourage the unsuccessful behaviors of fast, uncontrolled overeating, but they also drive and stimulate hunger. If you understand this and begin to choose differently, your personal control over your eating behavior will dramatically increase.

MEAL REPLACEMENTS: WHEN LIFE GETS BUSY

In the complex, jam-packed lives we create with kids, jobs, parents, spouses, friends, church, volunteer activities, and other demands, there is often precious little time to think about mapping out nutritious meals every day of the week. On those days when you feel worn to an absolute frazzle, even a salad will take too long to fix. For many of you, it becomes so much easier to grab something to eat and go—even if what you "grab and go" with is a low-response cost food that is certain to sabotage your compliance and suck you back in to a vicious overeating cycle.

If this accurately describes your life, at least at vulnerable, high-risk times, then there is another weight-management tool to consider that can stop you from giving in to your negative momentum: meal replacement beverages and bars. These are supplemental foods formulated with a balanced distribution of nutrients, including protein, a combination of carbohydrate sources, vitamins, minerals, and other natural, high-yield ingredients. Although nothing truly replaces a meal of real food, these energy-controlled products provide rounded nutrition that can fill in substantial nutritional gaps and keep you from straying when you are tired, busy, or overcommitted.

Thus it is an effective nutritional strategy, and indeed a good idea, to use meal replacements to substitute for a meal when you are time-pressed and literally may not have time to prepare or eat breakfast, lunch, or dinner, or as an occasional between-meal snack. I say "occasional" because many meal replacers pack in excess of 300 calories, and that's too much food energy for a snack.

But you do live in the real world, and if you do have to "grab and go," grab a healthy alternative and not some low-response cost, low-yield junk food. Look for meal replacements that meet specific nutritional and metabolic standards. There are many such products that meet the test, and the benefits are numerous:

Weight Control. Current nutritional wisdom tells us that eating several meals throughout the day (three regular meals and two snacks) helps stabilize blood sugar to control food cravings, and maintains a higher metabolic rate for a fat-reducing effect. Substituting meal replacements for regular snacks increases your meal frequency and provides access to these benefits.

Weight Maintenance. Meal replacements, when used sensibly to replace several meals a week as part of a long-term weight-maintenance strategy, will automatically reduce your caloric intake and prevent rebound pounds from returning and piling back on. Simply controlling your intake at one meal with a meal replacement, several times a week, is enough to keep your weight from returning—so say a number of weight-maintenance studies.

Behavioral Control of Eating. There is a significant behavioral aspect to having meal replacement products available. The very sight of meal replacements in places like your refrigerator, kitchen cabinet, purse, or gym bag can serve as a positive visual cue, a daily reminder, to not overindulge in foods or snacks you shouldn't choose, and to select a healthier alternative—the meal replacement bar or beverage—instead.

Exercise Recovery. These products are biochemically valuable following a workout. It is at this time when your muscles are begging to be refueled with certain nutrients, namely carbohydrates to replace lost muscle energy and protein for tissue repair, both of which can be readily supplied by meal replacements.

I've included some important guidelines in the box on page 178 for you to follow in selecting from the choices available.

I am, of course, not advocating that you use these products for every single meal on a daily basis in order to crash down to your desired weight. Such thoughtless, careless nutrition will cancel out any progress you've made and set you up for more periods of frustrating ups and downs in your weight. The wisest and best use of any meal replacement will always be as a snack or as an occasional substitute for a regular meal.

When shopping for a meal replacement product, read labels and look for a product that is:

- Complete and balanced. This means that the product is formulated with an appropriate nutrient balance of protein, carbohydrate, and fat (a good rule of thumb is roughly 15 to 26 grams of protein, 14 to 30 grams of carbohydrates, and 2 to 8 grams of fat).

- Fortified with vitamins and minerals. Fortification with these nutrients can fill in nutritional gaps and help make up for what you may not be getting from food.

- Calorie-controlled. Reducing the amount of calories you eat is an important part of getting your weight under control. Select meal replacements that are low in calories, no more than 230 calories per serving, in order to help promote long-term weight control.

- High fiber. Choose products that are fiber-enriched, with 6 to 8 grams of added fiber. Fiber is a natural, beneficial component of food that offers numerous weight-control advantages. In fact, clinical research suggests that supplementing your diet with additional fiber at this level promotes weight loss.

- Low in added sugar. Take a close look at the amount of sugar listed on the Nutrition Facts portion of the label. Check to make sure that the number of grams of sugar is no more than half the total carbohydrate grams. Example: if a product contains 30 grams of sugar and 40 grams of total carbohydrates, then there is far too much sugar in that meal replacement.

WHAT ABOUT VITAMIN AND MINERAL SUPPLEMENTS?

While I am on the subject of supplements, I want to talk to you about a related matter: the decision to use vitamin and mineral supplements as a part of your overall efforts to improve your health and well-being.

The more I review the ever-expanding medical literature on the value of nutritional supplementation, the more I am convinced that just about everyone can benefit from adding supplements to their daily routine. The payoffs for health are undeniable and well-documented. Study after study shows that nutritional supplements—vitamins, minerals, herbs, and other food factors—can support good health and prevent illness. You should always rely on a variety of healthy foods for your essential nutrients. Don't take supplements as an excuse to eat thoughtlessly, skipping fruits and vegetables to load up on junk food. Supplements should never substitute for healthy eating. They are only a "supplement" to good nutrition, not a substitute.

Now let's consider in greater detail the case for adding supplements to your own nutrition. Maybe you're among the 40 percent of the U.S. population who already take supplements on a regular basis. If you are, and they are correct for your body type and are of high quality, that's great. Taking supplements can be a smart thing to do, for several reasons.

First, if you are overweight, then by definition, I know that you are malnourished. It's true: obesity—just like starvation—is a disease of malnutrition. As you read this, your initial reaction might be to wonder if I have gone nuts. But hear me out: you've been eating more calories than your body needs, and those calories have been in the form of high-fat foods, sugar-laden foods, refined foods—all stuff that is nutritionally bankrupt. You have not been eating enough foods rich in vitamins, minerals, fiber, and other healthful components, and you've shortchanged yourself nutritionally. So you see: obesity is a form of malnutrition brought on by excessive intake of the wrong kind of calories. Amazingly, there are as many obese people in the world as there are people suffering from starvation!

Second, those junk-food calories you've been bingeing on are flushing health-enhancing nutrients out of your system. When sugar and refined carbohydrates go in, chromium, zinc, magnesium, vitamin B_6, and folic acid go out. This means your vulnerability to certain nutritional deficiencies is huge.

Third, if you've come to this program fresh from a history of on-again, off-again dieting, you may have increased needs for specific nutrients. Here's why: by their very nature, most diets restrict something, whether it's carbohydrates, fats, or specific types of food. And with that restriction comes a trade-off: a potential shortfall of vitamins and minerals. Research, in fact, indicates that dieters have marginal deficiencies in vitamin A, vitamin E, beta-carotene, various B vitamins, and calcium. As a chronic dieter, you either don't eat enough or you don't eat balanced meals, and consequently, you're missing out on specific nutrients.

Fourth, your lifestyle can upset the nutritional apple cart in a big way. For example, smoking and exposure to secondhand smoke and environmental pollutants can rob your body of vitamin C, without your even knowing it. Drinking alcoholic beverages interferes with your body's use of various B complex vitamins. So ultimately, what you create for yourself through poor lifestyle habits is a critical shortage of many vital nutrients. Supplementation can go a long way toward improving this condition, especially while you work on changing your health-defeating behaviors.

Here are some action steps to help you:

1. Select a high-quality multiple vitamin–mineral formula that contains antioxidants, nutrients that help protect your body from disease at the cellular level. Most medical experts feel that a daily multiple vitamin–mineral supplement at 100 percent the Recommended Daily Intake (RDI), or sometimes higher, is perfectly safe. For optimum nutritional and metabolic support, the product you use should also supply 200 percent or more of the RDI for key B vitamins, including thiamin, riboflavin, niacin, vitamin B_6, folic acid, and vitamin B_{12}. Look for a product manufactured by a reputable, recognizable company.

2. Take your supplement with meals. You need a little bit of fat from protein or dairy products to help your body better absorb vitamins A, D, E, and K.

3. Consider taking single supplements of the following: vitamin C (200 to 500 milligrams a day), vitamin E (100 to 400 IUs a day), and calcium (500 to 1000 milligrams a day). Calcium supplementation is a must if you are a woman and want to protect the health of your bones.

4. Inform your physician and pharmacist that you are taking supplements, since some supplements may interfere with prescription medications.

WHAT TO EXPECT

Now, let's move on to talking about what you can expect as you use this key. Once you begin eating high-response cost, high-yield foods, you will chalk up big weight losses that last because you'll be eating real food and highly nutritious foods. As you eat this way, making commonsense choices, day after day, week after week, month after month, expect to feel significant improvements in your weight, your energy level, and your mental outlook. I know this firsthand, because these are the results I've personally seen in so many of the overweight people I've counseled over my career.

With this approach to nutrition, your body uses more calories for energy than for fat storage. This is because high-response cost, high-yield foods are low in fat, sugar, and refined carbohydrates. Why is this important? It is well established that a major dietary determinant of obesity is consuming too many calories without burning them off, particularly in the guise of high-fat foods, sugary foods, highly processed foods, and other low-response cost foods. Overweight people simply eat more calories, more fat, and more carbohydrates than normal-weight people do. So if you continue to overeat, taking in more calories than your body can expend, then expect to get so big that you'll have to sit down in shifts. On the other hand, by avoiding this stuff and getting back in touch with how much you really need to eat, you'll gain a tremendous edge in managing your weight.

As you begin to reduce your intake of low-response cost, low-yield foods and eat more wholesome, high-response cost foods in the amount your body needs for optimum functioning, you will be amazed by how much stamina you suddenly have. Your mind will be sharper and more alert because it is not drugged up on junk foods, and your emotions will stabilize and be more positive because you are no longer caught up in a cycle of self-condemnation over your destructive eating patterns.

Finally, this isn't something you "go on and off." One reason you've strayed off diets in the past is because you ate from a limited, ho hum list of foods that soon became boring, and certainly unrealistic to eat forever. So you gave up and went back to whatever you wanted to eat. By contrast, on this plan, you'll choose a variety of real foods that are eaten in the real world, allowing you to live normally, stay the course, and pare off those all-too-visible extra pounds.

THE HIGH-RESPONSE COST, HIGH-YIELD FOOD PLAN: ACTION STEPS THROUGH THE DOOR TO FOOD CONTROL

There has been and will continue to be a raging controversy in nutrition about the "best" proportion of major nutrients for weight loss. The controversy centers around whether your diet should be high-carbohydrate, low-carbohydrate, low-fat, high-fat, or high-protein. I've read the diet books, I've listened to the diet gurus debate this ad nauseam, about who is right and who is wrong; meanwhile people like you who want to manage their weight just sit there thinking, what's the real deal?

Well, the real deal is none of the above. The real deal for weight loss and weight control is moderation across the board—moderate carbohydrates, moderate protein, and moderate fat, and this current, accurate information comes straight from nutritional scientists, not from weight loss gurus or food faddists. That being the truth of the matter, the High-Response Cost, High-Yield Food Plan provides moderate amounts of these nutrients, and moderate amounts are what make this plan livable.

It is built around a huge number of food choices, and supplies sufficient nutrition for weight control and good health. Organized into an easy-to-remember system of eating, its foods promote behavioral control, weight loss, and good health.

You will plan your nutrition around:

- **High-response cost, high-yield proteins.** Foods such as meats, fish, poultry, dairy products, and protein substitutes furnish protein for building and repairing the body. Examples of protein foods to choose are:

Fish and shellfish
Lean cuts of meat
    Beef
    Lamb
    Pork
    Veal
Poultry
    Chicken
    Turkey
Plant proteins
    Legumes
    Textured vegetable protein
    Soymilk
    Tofu
Eggs or egg whites
Low-fat dairy products
    Reduced-fat cheese
    Skim milk
    1% milk
    Low-fat cottage cheese
    Part-skim ricotta cheese
    Sugar-free yogurt

See Appendix B for a more extensive list of foods.

Each day, have:

- 3 servings of protein

- 2 servings of low-fat dairy products

- **High-response cost, high-yield carbohydrates.** Carbohydrates are energy foods, and your choices here are broad:

Fruits
Vegetables
Grains
Whole-grain breads
Cereals
Starchy vegetables

(See Appendix B.)

Each day, have:

- 2 to 3 servings of starches (breads, grains, cereals, or starchy vegetables)

- 2 fruits

- 4 servings of vegetables

- **High-response cost, high-yield fats.** Although you should use them sparingly, certain fats are included as high-response cost, high-yield foods. The reason is that there are a number of beneficial fats, and these are abundant in:

Vegetable oils
    Olive oil
    Canola oil
    Flaxseed oil
Fish
Nuts
Seeds

Nutritionally, these fats, in the right amounts, are protective against heart disease, blood sugar disorders, skin and joint problems, and many other illnesses.

Each day, have:

- 1 serving of fat

With this in mind, let's turn to the specifics of the plan—and look at how to start planning your meals.

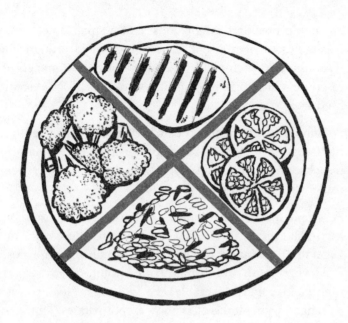

STEP ONE: DESIGN YOUR PLATE USING THE HIGH-RESPONSE COST, HIGH-YIELD FOOD LISTS

If you hate counting calories, adding up points, calculating carbohydrate or fat grams, multiplying nutrient percentages, and having to remember confusing details about food groups, then you will love what I am going to show you about meal planning. All you have to do is take out a dinner plate and mentally divide it into four sections, or quadrants.

At each meal, fill one section with a protein, another section with a starch, and the remaining two sections with vegetables or a vegetable and a fruit. Another way to look at this is that one-fourth of your food comes from protein, one-fourth from starch, and the rest (half of your plate) comes from low-calorie, high-fiber plant-based foods, including fruits and vegetables.

This is a system of meal planning I have always used when counseling overweight patients, and it is widely used by dietitians and health organizations to simplify mealtime nutrition. Proportioned in this manner, these foods form the foundation of your daily meals. You can use this system at every meal. For example:

- A sample breakfast might consist of a small omelet filled with vegetables (a high-response cost, high-yield protein and high-response cost, high-yield vegetables); a halved grapefruit (high-response cost, high-yield fruit); and grits (high-response cost, high-yield starch).

- A sample lunch might consist of salmon (high-response cost, high-yield protein); a salad of lettuce and tomatoes (high-response cost, high-yield vegetables); and brown rice (high-response cost, high-yield grain).

- A sample dinner might consist of roast beef (high-response cost, high-yield protein); green beans (high-response cost, high-yield vegetable); steamed yellow squash (high-response cost, high-yield vegetable); and a small baked potato (high-response cost, high-yield starchy vegetable). For greater fat loss, you may wish to reduce your intake of starchy carbohydrates, and you can do this easily by designing one-fourth of your plate with a high-response cost, high-yield protein, and the remaining three sections with high-response cost, high-yield vegetables (omitting the starch). A slight reduction in starch intake is known to help your body burn fat.

As for fats, the guidelines are simple, too. Have a tablespoon a day of high-response cost, high-yield fats or oils, or if the fat is a re-duced-calorie product, enjoy two tablespoons a day.

For snacks, choose mostly high-response cost fruits or vegetables, high-response cost milk products or, occasionally, meal replacement bars or beverages. Meal replacement beverages, which are available in ready-to-drink cans or powders that can be mixed with milk, can be used as your milk product allotment. Remember, allow yourself two to three fruits a day and two milk products a day.

STEP TWO: MANAGE YOUR PORTIONS

When using the divided-plate system for meal planning, there is the temptation to cheat, piling your portions as high as you can on your plate. That's why you do need to exercise additional portion control. That way, you don't eat too much or too little; instead you supply your body with exactly the amount that it requires. Please understand something here: I am not going to tell you to equip your kitchen with extra measuring spoons, measuring cups, and food scales, and begin measuring and weighing every morsel or tidbit before you eat. This is the wrong approach. I want you to keep your focus where it belongs, on nonfood-related activities, as much as you can.

When my friend and business partner Gary Dobbs decided to go on a diet a few years ago, the program he chose required that food portions be religiously weighed and measured. So for breakfast, lunch, dinner, and even snacks, Gary was forced to preoccupy himself with spooning vegetables into measuring cups, weighing chicken breasts on tiny food scales, counting out diet crackers, and taking so many dry measures, liquid measures, and volume measures that you would have thought he was the local weights and measures department. Gary told me in frustration: "With this diet, you're handling food all day. I'm counting this, and I'm counting that. I'm hauling food around with me all day in plastic tubs, and all I think about is eating. I'm jacking with food all the time, and I'm totally fixated on it!"

It became a cumbersome obsession to him, and this is where such rigid, legalistic diet programs can cause real trouble. Let me ask you this: you know that for recovery, alcoholics must abstain from liquor. But what if an alcoholic, fresh out of a substance abuse program, were placed in circumstances in which he was required to handle booze all day? I don't have to tell you what would happen, do I? If you are trying to control your intake of a substance, even if that substance is food, you have to get your focus off it, or you'll only be fueling your obsession.

Unless you are wired up with some kind of weird overly analytical brain parts that most of us don't have and take pleasure in weighing and measuring food, you do not have to go to these extremes. There are creative, super-simple selection devices that allow you to judge your portion sizes without having to handle measuring utensils and food scales all day long. All you have to do is picture portions of food relative to the size of your hand, or to a tennis ball. For example:

- A serving of meat, fish, or poultry should be about the size of the palm of your hand.

- Your fruit and vegetable servings should be about the size of your hand when it is cupped, or about the size of a tennis ball. (The volume of a tennis ball actually equals one half cup, considered the standard for one serving of fruits or vegetables.) Same for a serving of cottage cheese, rice, pasta, cereal, or starchy vegetables.

- Whenever you need a cupful of some food such as milk or yogurt, a serving the size of a fist or two tennis balls is about the right amount.

- A slice of bread, one small roll, or a half a bagel or bun counts as one serving.

- A serving of sandwich cheese is one slice.

- As for fats and oil or nuts and seeds, a reasonable serving is about the size of your thumb (or half your thumb if you've got big fingers).

If you eat out frequently, you can use these measures, along with the divided-plate system, to judge your portion sizes. (After all, you always have your hands with you, and who would take measuring utensils to a restaurant, anyway?) Using these measures when you dine out gives you more personal control, too, since restaurant portions are usually larger than the standard serving sizes you need for managing your weight. For instance, a baked potato at some restaurants is not actually one serving; it's more like two or three.

Whether you use this measuring system or some other, portion management can be a liberating factor in your life since it frees you from the anxiety of figuring out how much is enough. The amount of food you eat is no longer an exaggeration of your actual requirements, but is exactly what your body needs. And once you get the hang of it, portion management becomes something you do without even thinking about it.

STEP THREE: PLAN YOUR MEALS

For you to regain even greater control over food, you must make a food plan, then implement it. By food plan, I mean that you commit to paper exactly what you plan to eat each day, then eat only the foods on that list. The significance of having a well-planned food strategy is that it frees you from making last-minute decisions about what to eat, and prevents you from caving in to sudden impulses to overeat. Planning your eating in advance eliminates any doubt about what you will eat and removes your fear of losing control. No longer do you have to rely on the fickle emotion of willpower to keep you from eating what you know you shouldn't. Your food plan sustains your commitment in the absence of emotional energy.

When you plan, do so a day at a time and allow for three meals and at least two snacks. If you start your day with this strategy, with your foods and preferences outlined ahead of time, you guarantee the necessary forward movement that will help you stay the course, no matter what the situation.

While some of these guidelines on food planning are by no means new with regard to human functioning, the fact remains that you may be applying them to your weight-management efforts for the first time ever. Therein lies the difference. Up until now, you have been living in a reactive mode, responding arbitrarily on impulse to food temptations in your environment, and the more you reacted, the more unmanageable your weight became. With these planning tools, you can now program your eating behavior, rather than depend on willpower to see you through. As long as you rely on planning, strategy, and programming, not on willpower, it will be impossible for you not to lose weight.

To make all of this easy and workable for you, I've included a sample seven-day menu. Initially, you might be more comfortable following a prescribed menu because it removes so much of the iffy-ness involved in meal planning, plus helps ease the transition into new ways of eating. If you use my seven-day menu, feel free to switch meals around within these menus. For example, you can have a Day 1 breakfast any day of the week, or a Day 3 dinner on Day 7. With these menus, remember to rely on the divided-plate and portion-management tools I've provided for you.

As part of your daily meal planning, you must also plan for your fluid intake. Drink eight to ten glasses of pure water every day as your principal beverage. Water produces a feeling of fullness, plus helps enhance the physiological processes involved in fat metabolism and weight reduction. In fact, research has found that people struggling with obesity are notoriously poor water drinkers, hinting at a possible connection between obesity and water deficiency.

The Seven-Day High-Response Cost, High-Yield Food Plan

Day 1: Sunday

Breakfast:
Banana, oat bran (cooked), low-fat milk, coffee or tea

Snack:
Apple, meal replacement beverage

Lunch:
Tuna, vegetable soup, salad greens and sliced tomato, whole-wheat roll (medium), reduced-fat salad dressing

Snack:
Orange

Dinner:
Sirloin steak, baked potato with fat-free sour cream, broccoli, green beans

Day 2: Monday

Breakfast:
Raspberries (or other seasonal fresh fruit), multigrain bread (1 slice), egg (poached), coffee or tea

Snack:
Low-fat milk or sugar-free yogurt, fresh fruit

Lunch:
Low-fat cottage cheese, salad vegetables, ½ cup unsweetened pine-apple chunks, 2 tablespoons light fruit salad dressing

Snack:
Low-fat milk, orange

Dinner:
Turkey breast, stewed tomatoes, steamed summer squash, brown rice

Day 3: Tuesday

Breakfast:
Grapefruit, vegetable omelet, grits, coffee or tea

Snack:
Pear, sugar-free yogurt

Lunch:
Chili (meat and beans), cut up raw vegetables, reduced-fat ranch salad dressing for vegetables

Snack:
Smoothie: meal replacement beverage blended with frozen strawberries

Dinner:
Chicken breast, kale, small tossed salad, mashed sweet potatoes

Day 4: Wednesday

Breakfast:
Orange juice, sugar-free yogurt, bran muffin, coffee or tea

Snack:
Sugar-free coffee, vanilla, or lemon yogurt

Lunch:
Open-faced turkey sandwich: turkey breast and 1 slice reduced-fat Swiss cheese, whole-wheat bread, lettuce and tomato slices, reduced-fat mayonnaise

Snack:
Apple, meal replacement bar

Dinner:
Lean pork roast, spinach, small tossed salad with reduced-fat salad dressing, small baked potato

Day 5: Thursday

Breakfast:
Blueberries, high-fiber bran cereal, low-fat milk, coffee or tea

Snack:
Smoothie: low-fat or soy milk with frozen unsweetened peaches

Lunch:
Pita sandwich: canned salmon, whole-wheat pita, chopped celery, and reduced-fat mayonnaise; sliced tomato and raw carrots

Snack:
2 small apricots, meal replacement bar

Dinner:
Roasted Cornish game hen, winter squash, tossed salad, reduced-fat salad dressing

Day 6: Friday

Breakfast:
Grapefruit, bran muffin, egg (scrambled), coffee or tea

Snack:
Sugar-free yogurt, diced mango or other seasonal fresh fruit

Lunch:
Greek Salad: reduced-fat feta cheese, romaine lettuce, chopped onion, and reduced-fat salad dressing; whole-wheat bread, apple

Snack:
Low-fat milk or soy milk, meal replacement bar

Dinner:
Grilled swordfish, turnip greens, small fresh fruit salad, small baked yam

Day 7: Saturday

Breakfast:
Cantaloupe, sugar-free yogurt, small diameter (2½-inch) whole-wheat bagel, fat-free cream cheese, coffee or tea

Snack:
Smoothie: meal replacement beverage blended with a frozen banana

Lunch:
Steamed shrimp, cole slaw (made with reduced-fat cole slaw dressing), sliced tomato, cocktail sauce, whole-wheat roll

Snack:
Grapes

Dinner:
Lean ground beef, mixed vegetables, whole-wheat pasta with spaghetti sauce

Once you get the hang of how to eat using high-response cost foods in these mealtime proportions, you should map out your own

CHART 2. MY HIGH-RESPONSE COST, HIGH-YIELD FOOD PLAN MEAL PLANNER

MEAL	FOOD
Breakfast:	HRC/HY Fruit: HRC/HY Protein: HRC/HY Cereal or Bread: Other (Fat or Milk Product):
*Snack:	HRC/HY Milk: HRC/HY Fruit:
Lunch:	HRC/HY Protein: HRC/HY Vegetables: HRC/HY Grain, Bread, or Other Starch: Other:
*Snack:	HRC/HY Milk: HRC/HY Fruit:
Dinner:	HRC/HY Protein: HRC/HY Vegetables: HRC/HY Grain, Bread, or Other Starch: Other:

* *Meal replacement beverages or bars can be used for snacks, in addition to occasional meal substitutions.*

meals. For assistance, you can use the meal planner above to devise your meals each day.

As you prepare your foods, take advantage of seasonings which help your food taste better without having to add a lot of extra salt; fat-free condiments you can use to flavor your foods; and low-calorie foods such as lite soy sauce, Worcestershire sauce, tomato sauce catsup, salsa, hot sauce, horseradish, mustard, herbs, and spices. Other foods to use sensibly include bouillons and broths; sugar-free gelatins, jams, and jellies; and nonstick vegetable sprays. For additional planning guidelines, refer to the Do's and Don'ts at the end of this chapter.

STEP FIVE: STAY REAL AND STAY FLEXIBLE

As you become more familiar with the high-response cost, high-yield foods listed and recommended here, you may now be thinking that the plan looks restrictive. But let me reassure you that it is not; these lists and these strategies for meal planning are merely guidelines for ensuring the best possible results. Realize that while no food is really restricted, you must learn to refuse those foods you don't handle well, and choose better. Acknowledge which foods are a problem for you and learn how to control them.

To frame this important point in a real-world situation, allow me to share with you the story of a woman I once counseled, Colleen, who had for many years been struggling with binge eating and was at least 40 pounds overweight as a result of this behavior. When undergoing periods of distress, Colleen would consume huge quantities of food, and do so very rapidly, even if she was not hungry. She would habitually eat alone because she was mortified by her eating behavior. Following a binge, she would resume a diet, and with whatever diet she chose, there were food restrictions. Once she found herself in another stressful situation, Colleen would relapse into binge behavior, invariably bingeing on the very foods that were off-limits according to the diet she had been on. This was a vicious cycle, and Colleen was disgusted with herself and hated her body.

Prior to undergoing individual counseling, Colleen had pursued other avenues of therapeutic help, all to no avail. An unfortunate outcome of one of these attempts was that Colleen had been "brainwashed" to believe that, like an alcoholic she would be forever in a state of recovery—that she was a "recovering overeater." In effect, she was told that her condition was a permanent disability, that she would never be able to resume "normal eating." She bought into this line of reasoning. As a consequence, Colleen believed that she would never be able to enjoy a piece of pie, a slice of pizza, a dish of ice cream, that such foods were as dangerous as drugs or alcohol, and that if she ate them, she was a hopeless failure. Although she craved them, the fear she had attached to certain foods was overpowering, and the guilt she felt if she ate them was emotionally crippling. She beat up on herself relentlessly if she had so much as even a bite of one of these "off-limit" foods, and usually a bite would lead to a binge.

As I have said, food differs from alcohol or drugs in the following important regard: you can abstain 100 percent from alcohol and drugs, but you cannot abstain totally from food. Although the label of "recovering overeater" stemmed from good intentions, it communicated to Colleen that she lacked the capacity to deal in the "normal" world, with its huge variety of food and its many inducements to eat. The label boxed her into a sense of self-limitation involving her own power to exercise choices, and this had some awful mental and emotional consequences.

What Colleen had to do was begin to forge a new relationship with food. The realist in me knew that if she were ever going to escape that prison of fear and guilt associated with food and regain her power, Colleen would have to become desensitized to the foods she feared. One of my strategies for her was to have her eat a piece of cake or a piece of pie, at least once or twice a week. The required behavior was to eat only one piece, not the whole cake or pie. Her anxiety at this strategy initially went through the roof. (It may seem like cruel and unusual torture to you, but trust me, it is an undeniably powerful form of behavior therapy, and it works.)

To make a long story short, Colleen's fear of these foods gradually diminished with her exposure to them. She began to adopt a new, healthier attitude toward food—that certain foods were not inherently good or bad, but that they were foods to be eaten in smaller amounts or less frequently. Once she figured out what was best for her body, the choice of whether to eat a certain food depended on how she planned to use it in her diet: as everyday health-enhancing nutrition or as an occasional treat. That way, she met all of her body's needs for proper nutrition, without ever feeling deprived. With lifestyle changes such as becoming more active, Colleen dropped all of her 40 excess pounds—even while eating a piece of pie or cake once or twice a week—and more significantly, she became free of the fear and guilt that were formerly attached to certain foods.

What I want you to recognize is that when you or someone else, or even some diet, tells you that you can't have certain foods, expect your desire for them to intensify. People by nature want what they can't have; so you recognize the futility of food restrictions. For this reason, I am going to go against the grain of conventional diet wisdom and tell you to not cross any food off your list, unless it is a problem for you. I am not going to tell you that you cannot eat this or that. In fact, no particular food must necessarily be included or avoided.

So as you follow my High-Response Cost, High-Yield Food Plan, please stay flexible. Do not fixate on whether you ate the right number of servings yesterday, or whether you dished out the right portion size at dinner. If you want to eat cake and ice cream at your child's birthday party, then by all means, have it. Obsessing over what to eat and what not to eat will only sabotage your weight-control efforts, making it more difficult to lose weight. Your life should allow for some occasional treats, as long as you keep from bingeing or returning to a pattern of free-for-all eating.

Very important: never let one treat turn into an excuse for blowing your entire food plan. Many of you may still be locked in the grip of that all-or-nothing mentality we talked about in the first key. Your line of reasoning goes something like this: "I ate a bowl of ice cream. I blew it so I might as well eat the whole carton." Letting a treat or a little splurge be an excuse to go off on a protracted binge is so profoundly irrational that it will prevent you from ever gaining control over your weight. Sure, maybe you stumbled, but take that setback experience and use it as a catalyst to reaffirm your commitment and strengthen your resolve to do really, really better tomorrow.

If you do find yourself pining away for low-nourishment foods on which you formerly binged, you can select slenderizing substitutions for those foods: no-sugar ice cream for regular ice cream; chopped fresh vegetables with low-fat dip for the usual high-fat chips and dip; or fresh or dried fruit to satisfy a craving for candy. By opting for healthier substitutes that you have on hand, you will be able to manage the craving without giving in to it.

You can use the High-Response Cost, High-Yield Food Plan to maintain your new healthy weight for life. With your knowledge and understanding of how food works behaviorally and physiologically, you now have the tools to keep your weight under control and your health in balance. While maintaining your goal weight, for example, you may want to increase your nutrient intake slightly. For example, you may wish to add another fruit or milk serving to your daily menu, an extra serving of a high-response, high-yield starch (especially if you have become more physically active), or a small serving of some low-sugar, low-fat ice cream for dessert. Monitor your weight on the

HIGH-RESPONSE COST,
HIGH-YIELD FOOD PLAN DO'S AND DON'TS

High-Response Cost, High-Yield Food Plan Do's

Vary your food plan by eating an assortment of different foods. This helps assure that you get all the nutrients you need.

Eat at least two to three servings of fish a week in order to obtain the healthy fats that are abundant in seafood.

Eat at least one vitamin C-rich fruit a day. Examples include citrus fruits, citrus juices, strawberries, and cantaloupe.

Eat fruits and vegetables rich in vitamin A and beta-carotene most days of the week. These include apricots, carrots, and sweet potatoes—any orange, yellow, or red food, really.

Include plenty of high-fiber foods in your menus each day. Legumes (beans and lentils), fruits, vegetables, and whole grains are among the foods most plentiful in fiber.

Eat your foods at a slow, leisurely pace.

Use low calorie cookbooks to create varied and healthy meals, or rework favorite family recipes into reduced-calorie versions.

Shake the salt habit. Season your foods with herbs and spices in order to cut down on the amount of salt you use.

Drink eight to ten glasses of pure water a day.

High-Response Cost, High Yield Food Plan Don'ts

Do not eat sugar or sweets, or at least limit them to an occasional splurge.

Do not eat unhealthy fats, or at least try to limit them. These include saturated fats, found primarily in fatty animal products; tropical oils such as coconut oil and palm kernel oil; and "hydrogenated fats," a man-made fat containing unhealthy substances

(continued on next page)

called trans fatty acids, found in stick margarine, vegetable short-ening, and many commercially baked products.

Do not slather bread, rolls, and other foods with too much butter or margarine; avoid dishes such as tuna salad that have more mayonnaise than they do tuna and other ingredients.

Do not skip meals.

Do not eat after 7 or 8 P.M. at night. (Food eaten late in the evening is metabolized too slowly overnight and has a tendency to be stored easily as body fat.)

Don't eat more than three whole eggs a week if you have been diagnosed with heart disease.

scales, and when you see a gain, do a course correction. Return to the High-Response Cost, High-Yield Food Plan until you restabilize at your goal weight. If you manage your nutrition along with all the other steps, tools, and programming set forth in this book, it will be amazingly easy to maintain your weight loss.

When I counseled my overweight patients who had triumphantly reached their goal weight, this was the advice I always gave them as they prepared to face the future: you can eat any food you want, in reasonable quantities, some of the time. It's simply a question of how much and how often. But do go on alert that there are foods—low-response cost, low-yield foods—that are so behaviorally dangerous and nutritionally toxic because of their high sugar and refined carbo-hydrate content, that overeating them will result in the unhealthy, unwanted consequences of weight gain.

I will tell you, as I told them: never lose sight of the fact that if you frequently choose foods that are fattening and unhealthy or that you do not handle well, you will get inferior results and stay over-weight. If you choose foods that are wholesome and healthy, you will get superior results. The better your food choices, the better the re-sults. You know your goals: it's up to you to recognize which food choices support those goals and which do not.

9

Key Six:
Intentional Exercise
Unlock the Door to Body Control

*You have to stay in shape. My grandmother, she
started walking five miles a day when she was sixty.
She's ninety-seven today and we don't know where
the hell she is.*
—ELLEN DEGENERES

KEY #6: INTENTIONAL EXERCISE.

Prioritize exercise in your life. It is just too powerful a fat fighter for
you not to have it on your side. There is absolutely no way you can
control your weight for a lifetime without it.

This key is very straightforward: regular, intentional exercise is a
big deal, a huge deal. It unlocks the door to *body control*—a state of
fitness in which your body is metabolically geared for losing weight
and keeping it off, and is flowing with energy and vitality.

A common denominator among people who successfully manage
their weight and stay fit is that they exercise as a matter of habit.
Failure to put exercise at the top of your priority list, or leaving it off
the list altogether, is a deal breaker, because you're cheating yourself
not just out of a way to shed the necessary pounds, but also a way to
stabilize a normal weight and stay healthy for a lifetime. There will
be a huge difference between how you are now living and how you
will be living if you start prioritizing exercise in your life. Approach
this key with the most intense commitment, direction, and urgency
you can muster. Intend to master it. Your mission is to overcome the

inertia you now have and replace it with the forward momentum and direction you want. If you just jingle this key around in your pocket, you will never get what you want. To really get your weight under control, you must stop living like a lazy slug. Really managing your weight means that you will start requiring more of yourself in this important category of behavior.

Having said that, I am all too well aware that statistically, 66 percent of all Americans do not exercise. Perhaps right now you're among them. Perhaps you are still avoiding making the move to exercise. Perhaps you come home from work every day and crawl onto your couch like a slug on a stone and just sit there. Don't do that. Beginning today, please don't do that. While comfortable, that sort of nonreaching, inactive lifestyle can be more than inert, it's a choice that will keep you from ever getting your weight under control. Either you get this, or you don't, and I want you to be in the group that gets it.

Some of the most fit, in-shape people I have ever encountered were "once-and-former fatties" who overcame their weight challenges by making just one simple decision, and that decision was to become more active. In every case, this decision proved to be the beginning of a well-managed weight-control program and a healthy, well-managed life. Holly was one such person. Here is her story.

"I still carry this photo in my wallet," Holly told me, pointing to a picture of herself taken many years ago with her husband, Bob. "It's to remind me of how I used to look, 100 pounds ago."

Holly, 31, was a participant in one of my life skills seminars several years ago. It was difficult to believe that the person in the photograph—a very overweight girl swathed in a tent-like dress—and the trim, toned woman in the third row of the seminar were one and the same. But they were.

At the seminar, Holly related a story of great inspirational power. At barely 5 feet, 3 inches, she had not always been overweight, although she had steadily gained weight in the early years of her marriage when the couple hit some rough financial waters. Bob was laid off from his job as a human resources assistant after his employer was forced to cut back due to declining orders. The hard times continued, with Bob in and out of different jobs for about five years. During this period of time, Holly worked two management jobs in order to scrape by.

Emotionally stressed and physically drained, Holly began coping with the couple's budgetary challenges by eating ever-increasing amounts of food. Eventually, she became so addicted to food as an escape hatch from the financial distress that the overeating absolutely controlled her. Holly was spiraling downward, with no bottom in sight.

Life and money began to stabilize when Bob found employment at a company that offered more promise and security. But Holly, stuck in old patterns, was still a slave to food, and the pounds just kept piling on. At her heaviest, she pushed the scale up to 220. "I felt like the Goodyear blimp," she confessed. As time went on, Holly's weight began to cause serious health problems. The more she gained, the more lethargic she became. She had trouble breathing due to the strain of her weight on her heart and lungs. It was easier to sit than to stand.

The turning point came when Holly and Bob wanted to start a family, but their doctor warned that it was out of the question until she lost weight. Holly was told in no uncertain terms that her obesity could lead to miscarriage, and even if she carried a baby full term, she could put herself at risk for high blood pressure, infection, problems delivering a child, and other potentially serious complications.

Holly was shocked and scared. One day in the supermarket, she ran into an old friend from high school whom she had not seen in years. The friend remarked innocently, "When's your baby due?" Holly, crushed to the core, fled the store in tears.

At that very crucial point in her life, Holly had two choices: remain in bondage to food or break free from her obsession with food and the incapacitating effects of overeating. Wisely, she chose the latter, determined to change her style of living. No more eating mindlessly all day, no more slumping in the recliner, no more of the same, not ever again.

That very same day, Holly went for a walk. Barely a few steps out the door, she wanted to turn back, because her breathing was so labored. With every step, her thighs rubbed against each other, chafing her skin and causing huge patches of redness. It hurt just to move.

But she kept going and made it around her block. Every day afterward, she walked a little more, although her walks were slow and still painful. The more Holly walked, the less hold food had over her, and she began to eat more nutritiously. In less than a year, she had lost 50 pounds. The triumph gave her enough of a boost to join a gym where she learned to lift weights. By the end of two years, Holly was jogging several times a week and working out with weights three times a week. In her second year of exercising, she shed another 50 pounds and reached her goal weight of 115 pounds.

That was also the year Holly became pregnant. Her delivery went without incident, and she gave birth to a very healthy baby boy. The small amount of weight she gained while pregnant melted off, because her already-fit body was physiologically geared for maintaining a normal weight.

There is more than one happy ending to this story: Holly became a personal trainer at the gym where she worked out, helping others obtain what seems so elusive at first but is well within reach when you stretch yourself just a little farther each day. Holly is an inspiration to all, especially when she shares that picture of her former self.

Having been introduced to Holly and hearing her story, perhaps you understand that not much about your body, your weight, your appearance, or the way you feel will bring lasting change until you get off your duff and get moving. So please: don't push exercise to the side and ignore it. Please don't.

EXERCISE AUDIT

Let's take a break here and assess your current level of activity. The following audit asks you to give your best estimate of how often you perform various activities. You will use the information you glean to propel yourself to a new level of personal fitness. Be extremely frank in your responses.

PART A: MODERATE ACTIVITIES

"Moderate" activities are defined as those that expend approximately 200 calories an hour. These calories can accrue and be cumulative. For example, if you do housework for 20 minutes, three times a week, you've accrued one hour of activity and have burned 200 calories.

There is some clinical evidence that moderate activities, performed regularly throughout your week, can be helpful in weight control and may be protective against heart disease.

To assess your level of moderate activity, place a checkmark beside any of the following activities you participate in each week.

1. Climbing stairs rather than take an escalator or elevator for an accumulated one hour a week.

2. Parking farther away from your destination in order to increase your walking for an accumulated one hour a week.

3. Walking for pleasure (not exercise) at least one hour a week.

4. Moderate on-the-job activities (e.g., stocking shelves, moving materials, lifting objects) for an accumulated one hour a week.

5. Moderate yard work (mowing the lawn without a rider mower, digging, etc.) for an accumulated one hour a week.

6. Moderate housework (scrubbing floors, sweeping floors, washing windows) for an accumulated one hour a week.

Scoring for Part A:

Give yourself one point for each activity you checked. If your score is three or less, then your moderate activity level is well below the norm. You're not burning enough energy in your daily activities to make any significant differences in your health. If your score is four or higher, this level of moderate activity is good and does count partially toward effective weight management.

PART B: VIGOROUS ACTIVITIES

"Vigorous" activities burn 350 calories or more an hour. When performed at least three hours a week, these activities promote fat loss and greatly reduce your risk of heart disease.

To assess your level of vigorous activity, place a checkmark beside any of the following activities you perform each week.

1. Brisk walking, jogging, running, biking, or swimming at least two to three hours a week. (Aerobic exercise machines such as treadmills and stationary bicycles count here.)

2. Participating in an aerobic dance class at least two to three hours a week.

3. Participating in calisthenics or general exercise at least two to three hours a week.

4. Playing strenuous racquet sports (singles tennis, racquetball, handball, or squash) at least two to three hours a week.

5. Playing other strenuous sports (basketball, volleyball, backpacking, martial arts, skiing, etc.) at least two to three hours a week.

6. Lifting weights at least two to three hours a week.

Scoring for Part B:

Again, give yourself one point for each activity you marked. If your score here is zero, this means that either you're doing none of these activities or you're not performing them for a long enough duration to make a difference in your weight and your health. For each activity you checked, you're burning at least 700 to 1,000 additional calories a week, maybe more, depending on your level of effort. So a score of one indicates that you're definitely on the right track, expending enough exercise calories to spark metabolic changes that will enhance weight loss. A score of two or higher is even better and means you can lose about a half a pound of fat a week, provided you don't overindulge on too much food. Further, research tells us that people who burn up 2,000 calories a week can slash their risk of heart disease in half. If you scored three or higher, all the better. You're actively burning fat, at the rate of approximately one pound per week.

OVERALL INTERPRETATION:

The bottom line here is that you should be performing at least three to four hours a week of moderate activity and at least two to three hours a week of vigorous activity. That is the minimum requirement. If you're doing anything less, then you're not active enough. You need to jack it up and discipline your activity level toward having a fitter, healthier body.

THE POWERFUL PAYOFFS OF EXERCISE

The fact that your weight has been reeling out of control tells me that you have for too long been suffering from an imbalance between the amount of food you eat and the rate at which you burn that food for energy. You have been eating more than your body could use, so the overload was stored as fat, and you became overweight as a result. Exercising, in addition to moderating the quantity of food you eat, is an important, necessary way to restore your body's energy balance. Exercise burns calories; in fact, you can automatically lose a pound of fat in just five to ten exercise sessions, provided you do not take in a surplus of calories. Exercise also accelerates your metabolism, the physiological process that converts food into energy, so that you burn up more calories even at rest.

There's something else at work, too: food behavior and exercise behavior are highly interactive, with a powerful connection operating between the two. If you exercise on a regular basis, a rather amazing phenomenon occurs: practically without being aware of it, you'll begin to experience a weakening desire to overeat or binge. Your food behavior will begin to change almost automatically, and you'll make healthier food choices as a matter of routine. In fact, a growing catalogue of studies reveals that regular exercisers just seem to naturally eat more fruit and vegetables than their inactive, couch potato counterparts do. No one knows for sure why this is true, but I am sure that the carryover effects of exercise are related to the positive sense of well being it produces. You feel better so you want to eat better.

We need to talk more about these positive payoffs of exercise, because living an active life gives you more power over your weight and your health than you can ever imagine. Look at the table on page 206 for a detailed breakdown of the physical and psychological benefits of exercise. Let these sink in. How could you not want these results?

My hope is that you'll want to start generating these results in

TABLE 6. BENEFITS OF EXERCISE

	EXERCISE ADVANTAGES
Physical	Reduced body fat
	Faster metabolism
	Greater proportion of body-defining muscle
	Shapelier figure (women); more chiseled physique (men)
	Improved appearance
	Easier-to-maintain weight loss
	Increased strength and endurance
	More energy
	Better flexibility and mobility
	Protection against bone loss and osteoporosis
	Stronger immunity and resistance to disease
	Greater cardiovascular fitness
	Reduced risk of diabetes
	Reduced risk of developing some cancers
	Less desire to smoke, use alcohol, or overeat
	Improved sex life
	Slowing down of the aging process
Psychological	Sharper mental alertness and concentration
	Relief of tension, stress, and anxiety
	Brighter mood, less depression
	Improved body image
	Greater self-esteem
	Improved self confidence
	Stronger sense of self-discipline

your own life right away. When you do, when you start exercising as a matter of habit, you take your physical and psychological health up to a whole new level of functioning. Right now, this might seem like an unbelievably steep hill you have to climb, but if you take it one step at a time, you'll love the outcome. You'll love that you don't have to work so hard to control your weight. You'll love what you start seeing in the mirror. And you'll love the inner strength and energy you have to perform at the very highest levels.

There's no better time than right now to get serious about exercise—no handy excuses, no telling yourself "it's easier not to." With its 620 muscles working in sync to move the 206 bones on your frame, your body was engineered to be active. Unless you use your muscles, your body will begin to decay like three-day-old bananas left on a countertop. The old saying "use it or lose it" is true of every part of your body, particularly your muscles.

As I have said many times, when you choose the behavior, you choose the consequences. Start affirmatively choosing to exercise in order to get the incredibly powerful consequences that flow from that behavior. When it comes to having an active lifestyle, now's the time to set the bar of performance for yourself at a record high level, then with tenacious determination, strive to leap over it. Demand nothing less than the best of yourself and for yourself as you take up a brand new, more active way of living.

ACTION STEPS THROUGH THE DOOR TO BODY CONTROL

As one who has worked with thousands of overweight people, I have observed that many people simply don't like to exercise. In fact, many of you out there can probably identify with a forty-five-year-old woman I once worked with who told me: "I hate exercise. I'm sorry, I'm not athletic. I don't like getting sweaty. I don't like working out. I've given it my best shot. But I just don't like it."

Sharon absolutely fit the description of a couch potato, to a tee. At the same time, she was honest enough to own up to the fact that there were certain things in life she didn't like to do, and exercise was obviously one of them. I explained to Sharon that although she didn't like exercise, it was something she needed to do. I encouraged her to come to grips with this, in order to avoid caving into her negative momentum. Fortunately, she was mature enough to admit that yes, she did need to become more physically active.

In working with Sharon, to further pry her out of her self-ordained physical laziness, I designed a very specific plan that was failure-proof, guaranteed, one that would radically change her weight and her lifestyle. I set up a contract with her that she would exercise three times a week, at the very minimum, and she agreed that she would give it a go for one month. And she did. She stuck it out. By the end of the contractual month, an inspiring change had come over Sharon. I remember her sitting in my office, energetic, enthusiastic, her eyes sparkling, telling me: "I never thought I'd say this, but I am beginning to really enjoy exercising. It has become a part of who I am. I'm proud of myself for making such a positive change in my lifestyle."

Wow—did you get that? Don't let what you just read fly over your head: Sharon moved from a position of hating exercise to disciplining herself enough to do it on a regular basis. She replaced her "I don't like it/I don't want to do it" attitude with a "yes I can do it" mind-set. How did that happen?

As Sharon did, to get from point A—hating exercise—to point B—making exercise a part of your lifestyle—you must connect some dots. This is a process that, along the way, requires pushing yourself to exercise, and allocating your time and energy to make it happen. That's what you have to do, and I am going to show you how. So that you have some idea of the roadmap you'll be following here, the dots connect like this:

> You must make exercise motivating, by choosing an activity or activities that you enjoy doing, and that you can do with a reasonable level of skill and mastery.
>
> You must set up your world in such a way that it easily allows you to pursue those activities on a regular basis, without interference. You must program yourself for exercise success.
>
> You must ramp up your exercise effort so that your body is physiologically capable of losing weight and counteracting weight gain. When you do this, you maximize your weight loss and your ability to keep your weight off permanently.
>
> The result, the ultimate outcome is that you can lay claim to most or all of the powerful and positive payoffs of exercise that I listed for you above, and keep your weight off for good.

You must move through this connection process as if your life depended on it; for a lot of you, it does. Your mission is to reverse the negative momentum you now have and get moving in a positive direction. Really changing your lifestyle with regard to exercise means that you will reorganize yourself and your life in such a way that it is absolutely impossible for you to fail. The famous advertising slogan from Nike sums it up best: "Just do it." To this I would add: Just do it, again and again and again. That's what we're about to do now. So if you're ready, let's just do it.

STEP ONE: MAKE IT MOTIVATING

For exercise to become a permanent fixture in your life, the activity or activities you pursue must have *reinforcing value* for you. In a nutshell, this means that you keep doing them because you like to do them, you can slot them conveniently into your lifestyle, and you derive emphatically positive payoffs, in the short term and in the long term, from doing those activities. When you do what you enjoy, the exercise becomes so very much easier. Liking an activity and getting positive payoffs from it become cues in themselves for performing that activity.

So the first meaningful connection in the process of becoming a lifelong exerciser is to identify an activity that appeals to you. You might have to experiment, trying out any number of different activities before you settle on the right one. Just don't give up, just don't throw in the towel. Find something you like to do, so much that you want to continue doing it for a lifetime.

The exercise you're considering must be something you are good at, have the physical ability and coordination to do, or believe you can master. It must be something you feel you can perform competently with a reasonable degree of skill, to realize positive results. In shrink talk, this is called *self-efficacy*, and it determines whether you will take on a new behavior, the amount of effort you'll expend on it, and how likely you are to stick with it in the face of difficulty and other barriers. In shorthand terms, self-efficacy describes a "can-do" spirit. The greater your self-efficacy in a chosen exercise, the more likely you are to stick with it and make it part of your life.

When thinking about which form of exercise to pursue, take your own physical limitations into account beforehand. If you cannot physically perform a certain exercise, there is no way you will build self-efficacy, and you should not even consider the activity in question as viable. Take me, for example. I have no sense of balance. If I try to stand on one foot, I keel over like a felled timber—so skiing, roller blading, or any activity that requires balance is out of the question for me.

Self-efficacy doesn't happen automatically; it has to build with time and practice. Suppose you decide that jogging interests you. At first, the prospect of jogging 30 minutes a day seems so out of reach that you want to give up before you've even hit the track running. Instead, break your jogging down into small steps; at first, perhaps, it is 10 minutes a day of jogging, then 15 minutes, then 20 minutes. Soon you're jogging 30 minutes or more daily, with so much enthusiasm and ability that maybe you start considering competing in a marathon.

So think through what might work for you. Maybe you enjoy competitive activities, including team sports. The following activities might be right for you:

- Any active team sport such as basketball or volleyball in which you are constantly on the move

- Tennis

- Racquetball

- Handball

- Golf (pulling your own cart)

- Martial arts

- Competitive endurance sports such as running or competing in marathons or triathlons

Or maybe you prefer exercising alone as opposed to group activity or team sports, following an organized routine, with specific exercises and measurable goals to attain. Activities that best suit you include:

- Strength training

- Exercise machines (treadmill, stair climber, stationary bicycle, etc.)

- Walking

- Jogging

- Running

- Swimming

- Hiking

- Biking

- Home exercising

Perhaps you enjoy working out with other people, particularly in exercise classes or in facilities where there are plenty of people. In addition, you enjoy working out with a partner. Some of the best exercise options for you might include:

- Any type of group exercise class (aerobic dance, for example)

- Strength training when accompanied by an exercise partner

- Group endurance activities (running clubs and biking clubs, for example)

You may be someone who prefers low-impact activities that emphasize flexibility and are conducted in a quiet atmosphere designed to bring about inner stillness. In addition, these activities may be appropriate for you right now if you have certain physical or medical limitations, and need a gentler form of exercise. Some options to consider:

- Yoga

- Pilates

- Tai chi

- Stretching

After thinking through all these options, perhaps you discovered that there are a number of activities that appeal to you, from sports to exercise classes to individual pursuits such as weight training. This is a good thing, because it means you can vary your activities to provide a change of pace and prevent boredom from settling in.

Bottom line: choose activities that appeal to you, that you feel you can perform with a reasonable degree of skill, then be patient enough with yourself to gain the requisite mastery. The reality that you're getting good at exercise, plus getting results from it, will reinforce your positive behavior. Once you have settled on some sort of physical exercise, the next step in the connection process is to program your lifestyle in such a way that it is impossible for you to avoid exercising.

STEP TWO: PROGRAM AN ACTIVE LIFESTYLE

Committing to exercise is another area of health behavior where you typically default to relying on willpower. As I've said many times already, willpower is unreliable emotional fuel that runs down, leaving you no better off than you were before. It works like this, and you know the story line, chapter and verse: come January 1, you don your seldom-worn jogging suit, sweats, or leotard and hit the pavement, pump iron, or sweat a few exercise classes, but by January 31, your willpower has snapped, and you've reclaimed couch potato status.

It's a familiar ritual, one you go through, time after time. Admit it, there's a terrific strain within you as you try to hold it all together. All that emotional steam, all that emotional energy you're expending is just adding to your trouble—burning you out, really. When you try to change out of sheer willpower, you're headed for certain failure. Sure, you need some "want to," but permanent success doesn't come from forcing yourself; it comes from programming yourself and your world to do better. That is how you accomplish what you really want to do.

Programming an active lifestyle means incorporating exercise into your day-to-day life so that you can do it with as few changes or disruptions in your routine as possible. You set your life up so that exercise is as normal and as routine as brushing your teeth.

Having said that, I am all too well aware that the number one excuse people give for not exercising is "I don't have time." Well, if that's your excuse, my question for you is "Do you have time *not* to exercise?" If you don't exercise, you are saying, in effect, that you have time to stay overweight and that you have time, at some point in your future, for a long, and still growing list of life-crippling, life-threatening diseases that exercise is known to prevent. If you don't have time for exercise, ask yourself if you have time for heart disease, stroke, cancer, or diabetes. If you don't exercise with some degree of regularity, you are making a decision to compromise your life quality, today and in the future.

Whenever I hear this overused excuse, I think of our longtime family friend, Anna. Anna, wife and mother of four lively school-aged children, leads the kind of on-the-go frenetic lifestyle that so many of us now take as normal. One minute she's at a teacher-parent conference, the next at a Little League game, later at church, serving on a volunteer committee. And so it goes, day after day, week after week.

Now you'd think Anna doesn't have a moment to call her own, much less exercise. Wrong.

Anna is a regular exerciser and has been for years. What's her secret?

She uses time that's already available. It's not that she doesn't have time—she does—she uses the time she already has.

Before each week starts, Anna checks her calendar to identify commitments involving her kids, always the week's priority. Once these are blocked out, she schedules the times when she can go to the gym, times that are already there. It's just a simple case of good planning.

And instead of considering exercise a grind she can't wait to finish, Anna considers it a part of her daily routine for life. And rather than take time away from her family, exercise actually improves her family life. It puts her in a better frame of mind, it makes her feel good about herself, and it improves her overall outlook—all attitudes that are emotionally nourishing for those with whom she's sharing her life.

So let's agree right now that you will schedule specific times during the week to exercise. Then I want you to protect that time just as you do your other important activities of daily living. For example, you would not even consider getting up in the morning and going to work without first getting dressed, doing your makeup, or combing your hair. You would never say, "I don't have time to style my hair so I will just wear my hot rollers to work," or "I don't have time to get dressed so I will wear my pajamas to the office." Making time for exercise, then protecting that time—that is what is required here if you expect to start losing weight and managing yourself in an empowering way. No matter how hectic your life is, no matter how chaotic your schedule, you can make time, even if it means working out to an exercise video while your kids are napping or otherwise occupied. Bottom line: no excuses. What matters if you are to succeed is that you make the time, and then you use the time.

Your decision to exercise must become so important that you are willing to carve out time in your schedule, several times a week, every week, to do it. That is exactly what I want you to do in this step: take out your calendar, Day-Timer, whatever you use to record appointments, and ink in times in which you will exercise, even if at first it is only twenty minutes of walking three times a week. My rule for you is this: keep those appointments just as you do your other appointments with your doctor, dentist, barber, or hair stylist. Let nothing interfere, absolutely nothing.

At first, exercising will bring on some pain and discomfort but this will subside as your brain counters these unpleasant feelings by producing natural chemicals called endorphins, which are messengers of the pleasure sensation. The more you exercise, the stronger these pleasurable sensations become. You might not like exercising at first, but keep at it, and before you know it, exercise will become the rule rather than the exception in your life. Remember that your weight and your overall health are sustained, positively or negatively, by the lifestyle and environment you have set up. Creating a new, physically active environment is critical to keeping your positive life momentum alive.

Planning and scheduling exercise is a programming tool essential to your success because it provides structure, so as not to leave exercise to your own trial-and-error methods. A good exercise program should be structured enough with time-protected exercise sessions so that it props you up and propels you forward during times when you don't feel like exercising. You can't miss your exercise session because it is already structured into your week. Scheduling exercise into your week is an important self-discipline in achieving permanent weight loss and control.

You may wish to program yourself for exercise success in other ways as well. One important move is to keep a workout diary that tallies up your achievements—the miles you've walked or jogged, the weights you've lifted, the exercise classes you've attended, or the number of times per week you participated in active sports. A personal recordkeeping program, maintained honestly, provides important feedback on your progress, keeps you "on task," and shows you, in black and white, the substantial progress you are making toward improved fitness. To assist you in this, I have included a Workout Diary in Appendix C that you can adapt or modify to suit your own needs. Additional exercise guidelines for success are listed at the end of this chapter.

Another critically important move is to program your environment in such a way to support your goals. There's no better example than Jacob, another person I worked with who initially hated exercise, considering it a drudge he preferred to put off. To make it as easy as possible, what he did was to set his exercise clothes out before he went to bed at night. Upon arising, Jacob would jump into those clothes and go for a 30-minute walk. He began to do this without fail, his clothes a constant reminder to stay with it, and before long, he was able to maintain this exercise program as part of his daily routine for life.

Similarly, another patient, Katrina, made tremendous changes simply by keeping a fresh set of workout clothes in her car and driving by a health spa every day on her route home from work. It was convenient enough that she could drop in after work, exercise, then head home. She rarely missed a workout because she had programmed herself strategically for a life of energy and activity.

Then there is Ted, who joined a lunchtime walking group at work. Every noon, at the designated lunch hour, Ted and several coworkers lace up their walking shoes and hoof it briskly around the factory where they work.

Each one of these people adjusted their lifestyles to make more room for exercise and to make it easy to exercise. They made their environments "exercise-friendly." You can do the same. Have cues or reminders in your environment—your exercise clothes in plain view, a treadmill by your desk, or a route home that takes you by your gym—to make it easy to fall into exercise with as little trouble as possible.

STEP THREE: "CONSEQUATE" YOUR EXERCISE BEHAVIOR

This step acknowledges that *contingency management* is often needed to support and reinforce productive but initially less pleasurable behaviors such as exercising. Contingency management is a way in which you can reward yourself, conditional upon performing a specific behavior first. It is based on an important behavioral premise that people will perform less pleasurable activities if they are the path of access to the more desirable activities.

To illustrate this concept in everyday terms, let me use an example every one of you who are parents will be familiar with: as is customary, your child has homework to do after school; as is just as customary, he is reluctant to do it. You tell your child, "You can watch your favorite TV program tonight, but only if you do your homework first." You have, in essence, made watching television contingent upon doing homework first. Watching TV is the incentive for your kid to do his homework. If he doesn't do his homework, there is a consequence: no TV.

In using contingency management (I bet you didn't realize how well you were practicing psychology!), you "consequated" your child's actions. You equated, or paired, two activities—one a less desirable behavior (doing homework) and the other his reward (watching TV). There was a consequence to doing or not doing the less desirable behavior. I am sure your own parents and grandparents used this technique when they told you, "You must eat your dinner before you go out and play." The beauty of contingency management is that it has the power to change the frequency of a behavior for the better by altering its consequences.

When I counseled chronically obese patients in my practice, I repeatedly used contingency management, particularly in motivating people to comply with the exercise programs I had established for them, and I would consequate their compliance with something they valued such as personal grooming. In one case, I was working with a group of men, who, if it weren't for lifting their forks to their mouths at mealtimes, would have never gotten any exercise. I mean, these guys were worst-case lazy. In Texas, we compare people like that to blisters: they show up after the work's all done. Anyway, you get the picture.

Here is what I did: I instructed them to have all of their shirts for work each week laundered, starched, pressed, and folded—but to keep those fresh shirts in lockers at the local YMCA, not at home. In order for them to dress for work—which they had to do, they couldn't go to work in their pajamas—they had to go to the Y to get their shirts. And while they were at the Y, they were required to exercise. Being able to dress for work was made contingent upon going to the Y in the morning and exercising while they were there. In other words, the message was: unless you first exercise at the Y (action), you cannot get dressed for work (consequence). I assigned a consequence to their actions, and it made a huge difference in their behavior. These guys—the laziest of the lazy—converted from confirmed couch potatoes to committed exercisers, and it transformed their lives and their health for the better.

So consequate your exercise behavior. Decide: what will it take? What type of contingency management will be the most effective in getting you to exercise? Don't think that there is any kind of contingency management that is insignificant; the key is to make it matter enough to you so that you feel motivated to pursue constructive behavioral changes. You might undertake several types of contingencies to help program yourself and change your behavior. For example: if you don't exercise in the morning, you can't comb your hair. Or, if you don't exercise, you don't put on makeup or take a shower. No contingency is too trivial for consideration.

Time out here: I bet you think you will "cheat" on this step and not really follow through with your contingencies. You might just give yourself an excuse or two to let yourself slide. You might just decide to surrender right now, bail out, and wave your white flag. Fine, but if you do, you will only be cheating yourself out of a chance to lose weight and achieve genuine health and well-being. Read this as though I am speaking directly to you: effective weight management demands that you require more of yourself in terms of personal integrity, honesty, and maturity. Get real enough with yourself to say,

"I'm mature and honest enough not to play mind games with myself."
It's true, you do have substantial challenges here, but once you commit to a new level of integrity and maturity, being true to your contingencies will be a matter of principle.

STEP FOUR: MONITOR YOUR PROGRESS

When it comes to exercising, some people move like they're dragging
an anchor. That won't get it done. In order to shift your exercise program into high gear, you've got to be able to determine your level of
progress. You have to have some way of knowing whether you are
working at a level that will help you lose all the pounds you want to
lose.

In an aerobic exercise program, one way to keep tabs on your
progress is to use a heartrate monitor. I find that this technology is a
great way to monitor my own exercise effort. If I don't use it, it's like
I'm idling in neutral, and I won't work my heart enough beats per
minute to make a difference. But by using a heartrate monitor, I'll
push myself to the upper boundaries of my heartrate range for my age.
A heartrate monitor keeps you accountable.

The costs of these devices are affordable; most are well under
$100. You can wear them like a wristwatch, and with some, you can
download the results into your computer to keep easy track of your
progress over time.

To calculate your target heartrate zone, subtract your age from
220. That's your Maximum Heart Rate (MHR), which is pretty hard
to achieve and maintain unless you're an Olympic athlete on compe-
tition day. You'll want to keep your pulse between 50 and 75 percent
of your MHR. Hitting at least 60 percent means you're having a good
workout and is a reasonable goal. When you can reach 75 a few times
a week, it indicates you've achieved really peak condition. Anything
below 50 percent is coasting, and you'd be better off timing yourself
with a calendar. Table 7 (page 219) shows the general ranges for
heartrate based on your age.

Once you've identified your number, strap on your heartrate
monitor, and as you work out, strive to keep your heartrate in your
zone, after warming up.

TABLE 7. TARGET HEARTRATES DURING EXERCISE

AGE	TARGET HEARTRATE ZONE IN BEATS PER MINUTE (50 TO 75% OF MAXIMUM)	MAXIMUM HEARTRATE
20	100–150	200
25	98–146	195
30	95–142	190
35	93–139	185
40	90–135	180
45	88–131	175
50	85–128	170
55	83–124	165
60	80–120	160
65	78–116	155
70	75–113	150
75	73–109	145
80	70–105	140

If you don't use a heartrate monitor, check your pulse by placing two fingers lightly on your wrist (on the side by your thumb) or on your neck at your carotid artery (do not press hard). Count the beats for 10 seconds and multiply by six.

STEP FIVE: MAXIMIZE YOUR WEIGHT LOSS

At the gym where we have a family membership, there's a familiar scene in the workout room: women draped in jewelry, their hair perfectly coifed, their color-coordinated warm-up suits crying at the seams. They stand around and socialize for forty minutes, step on the treadmill for a few minutes, lift some weights, then socialize some more. In two hours there, they don't get five minutes of exercise, and

I've never seen one of them break a sweat. Then there are the men who come in every day after work, put on their exercise clothes, and head for the stationary bikes, where they read the business section of the newspaper while pedaling snail's-pace slow. Even the most casual observer could pick up that these people are not exercising!

What I'm telling you here is that once you've got some positive momentum going—you're exercising at something you like and you're programming your world to help you stay with it—you've got to gradually ramp up to make your exercise meaningful in terms of losing weight and getting fit. Exercise physiologists generally recommend that if you are overweight or obese, you should gradually and eventually progress to exercising five hours a week.

As you shoot for this goal, you can't just go through the motions; you've got to put some oomph into your exercise. This means if you're taking a yoga class twice a week, maybe you ramp up to taking that class three or four times a week. This means if you're walking around the block two times, maybe it's time to circle the block five times. This means if you're walking without any problems, maybe you might want to pick up the pace and do some jogging. This means if you're doing the stair-climbing machine at your gym for aerobic exercise, it might be time to add a strength-building component such as weight training to your program.

For an even greater fat-burning boost from aerobic exercise, try shorter bursts—about five to ten minutes of heart-pumping activity, punctuated by five minutes of slower activity in order to lower your heartrate. For example: ten minutes of jogging, interspersed with five minutes of walking, and so forth, for a total of forty-five to sixty minutes of aerobic activity. This method of exercising has been validated in research to have tremendous fat-reduction effects.

I'm not saying, however, that you have to sweat pints or do huff-and-puff workouts until you're blue in the face. That may be okay for people who have exercised all their lives and haven't had to battle a weight problem, but it may not be okay for you, especially if you haven't exercised in a long time. In fact, if you jump into this with a go-to-extremes philosophy, you may wind up injuring yourself.

I'm talking about gradually letting yourself do more, and taking deliberate, progressive action to get there. Okay, maybe you're rationalizing right now that you can't, that you've never pushed this far or this much before. Don't let your *can't* get in the way of your *can*. You can do this. It's just that you haven't—yet. Choose to give yourself the chance.

When you do, when you push for more, you will achieve such a higher level of conditioning that you will feel better than you have ever felt. Don't get me wrong; I'm not talking about training for a marathon here. It's considered an intense effort if you're walking, jogging, running, and so forth fast and hard enough so that you can still carry on a conversation, but you are breathing a little faster. This means that your heartrate is in a good range for cardiovascular conditioning, and that you've reached a good target for fat-burning. With aerobic exercise at this level, you'll burn more fat, and you'll turn your heart into a stronger pump so that it beats less often but pumps more blood.

The other important recommendation for increasing the fat-burning value of exercise is to add some form of strength-developing activity such as weight training to your exercise schedule, at least twice to three times a week. This is a big, big deal in terms of weight control, so I am going to make a big deal out of it.

Weight training is an excellent way to give those unwanted pounds a speedier heave-ho. Yes, aerobic exercise such as walking or swimming and flexibility-enhancing exercises such as stretching or yoga are important—and there should be aerobic and flexibility components to your exercise program—but there are specific benefits that only weight training can bestow. Exercising with weights burns fat and preserves muscle while you're losing weight (nearly 100 percent of the weight you lose is pure fat if you weight train); it strengthens your muscles, joints, and bones; it decreases your insulin levels so that your body is in better hormonal balance; and it makes maintaining your weight loss a breeze. In fact, a number of just-published studies have found that weight training stands out as a proven lifestyle strategy for keeping excess weight off over the long term.

Weight training throws your metabolism into high gear so that you burn calories even at rest, without even trying. Each pound of body-firming muscle you add to your frame becomes a fat-incinerating furnace, allowing you to eat moderate amounts of food without worrying about gaining fat. Once you've rid yourself of the weight you set out to lose, that new muscle keeps your metabolism purring along, and as long as you keep working out with weights, you needn't fear ballooning back to your old size. You don't have to cut back on food so drastically, since the newfound muscle you've acquired is burning up calories so fast.

As you continue to exercise with weights, expect to see exciting changes in your body. You'll begin to look completely different from how you ever thought you could. Gone are your love handles, your spare tire, your doughy hips and thighs. In their place are a tight waistline, a firm butt, legs you don't have to hide under baggy clothes—in short, a younger-looking body and a younger-functioning body. You'll look better than you have in your entire life, and you'll feel at your absolute best.

Many of you women out there are saying, "That sounds great, but there is no way I'm going to lift weights. I'm big enough already, and I don't want to turn into the Incredible Hulk."

Warning! Red alert! This is old thinking and it is wrong thinking. As a woman, your hormonal profile (namely the lack of male hormones) will prevent you from ever hulking or bulking up, no matter how hard you work out. When you weight train, it's like taking a little chisel to your body. Off comes blubbery thigh fat, gone is the jiggly butt. There's muscular definition in your arms you never knew you had. You're firm all over, and smaller, and better proportioned, too. You'll feel so good about yourself and what you've accomplished that you'll decide that brownies, potato chips, and pizza just aren't worth it anymore.

Whether you're a man or a woman, you're going to be so much more successful at managing your weight if you will take up weight training as part of your exercise program. If you're new to weight training, it is important to understand and follow several basic guidelines:

- Get instruction from someone who is qualified to teach you proper lifting techniques, including how to use dumbbells, barbells, and exercise machines. This person could be a certified personal trainer or coach who has experience in this form of exercise. Most gyms and health spas have these people on staff, and their training services are usually free.

- Begin your workout with a warm-up such as five to ten minutes of light aerobic activity on a treadmill, stationary bike, or a few laps around a track.

- Use light weights at first—poundages that you can lift easily for twelve repetitions without straining. This will not only build strength and enhance muscle tone, it will also help condition your tendons, ligaments, and the connective tissue around your joints. Increase the amount you're lifting by one or two pounds at your next workout.

- In your workouts, target every muscle group: your legs, abdominals, chest, shoulders, back, and arms. All you'll need are just six to ten different exercises to thoroughly work your entire body. Repeat each exercise two to three times (that is, two to three "sets" of about eight to ten repetitions). This may take only thirty minutes of your time, too. Do your weight-training workout just two to three times a week, on nonconsecutive days in order to allow your muscles sufficient time to restore themselves.

A WORD TO BEGINNERS

If you're emerging from a state of couch potato-ness, without ever exercising regularly or at least not in a while, you'll need to break yourself in gently and gradually. You've got to build up a little at a time. Here's a suggested program to help you get in gear, with weekly goals to help program you for success.

Let your physician know that you plan to start an exercise program and get his or her okay. This is vitally important, particularly if you have chronic health problems such as heart disease or diabetes. If you're a man over forty or a woman over fifty and you plan to start an exercise program, consult your physician in order to rule out any existing health problems, as well. Chances are your physician will applaud your decision, since for most people, exercise is an important form of preventive medicine needed nearly every day.

As a parting shot, I don't want you to guess where I've been coming from: the more active you are, the better your results. If you put off exercising, let me remind you that your clock is ticking. If you re-

TABLE 8. SAMPLE EXERCISE PROGRAM FOR BEGINNERS.

A Sample Eight-Week Exercise Program for Beginning Exercisers	
Week One Goal	2 days of brisk walking or other aerobic activity, 20 minutes each; 1 weight training session
Week Two Goal	3 days of brisk walking, or other aerobic activity, 20 to 30 minutes each; 2 weight training sessions
Week Three Goal	4 days of brisk walking, or other aerobic activity, 30 minutes each; 2 weight training sessions
Week Four Goal	4 days of brisk walking, or other aerobic activity, 30 minutes each; 3 weight training sessions.
Week Five Goal	5 days of brisk walking, or other aerobic activity, 30 minutes each; 3 weight training sessions
Week Six Goal	5 days of brisk walking, or other aerobic activity, 30 to 45 minutes each, 3 weight training sessions
Week Seven Goal	6 days of brisk walking, or other aerobic activity, 30 to 45 minutes each; 3 weight training sessions
Week Eight Goal	6 days of brisk walking, or other aerobic activity, 45 to 60 minutes each; 3 weight training sessions.

main inactive, then days, weeks, months, and years will continue to be wasted: time that could and would have been amazing and significant in your life. But start today, and in a time span as brief as ten minutes into your workout, you will feel better, you will be energized, you will have a better frame of mind and outlook on what lies ahead. You've just got to make the move. If you don't, it becomes easier and easier to stagnate and stay dormant. Stop justifying your own inactivity and stop avoiding the challenge of change. Changing your lifestyle from inactive to active requires energy and commitment, but easy or hard, I'm telling you that you must do it. It's your weight, your health, and your life at stake.

EXERCISE STEPS TO SUCCESS

- For exercise, wear shoes with proper support. I'm talking about some good fitness shoes or running shoes, designed expressly for specific types of workouts. They provide better motion control, and cushion your impact against the floor or ground while you're working out. Those old, beat-up shoes you wear when mowing your lawn or doing yardwork won't cut it; they're an invitation to ankle, knee, and joint problems.

- Dress appropriately by wearing clothes that allow you to move comfortably and allow your body to breathe. Be sure to dress for the temperature, too. Wearing a sweat suit to help you lose weight is dangerous, since it can cause dehydration and possibly bring on collapse. It's a myth that sweat suits help you lose fat. The only thing lost is water—and energy, if you get dehydrated.

- Warm up your body correctly by increasing your body temperature, gradually and gently. This may involve slow pedaling on a stationary bicycle or light walking at a normal pace. You can then perform some light stretches for your muscles after your body has warmed up. A proper warm-up helps counteract postexercise soreness or injury.

- As important as warming up is cooling down after each exercise session. Your cooldown period should include several minutes of light stretching or walking.

- In addition to a heartrate monitor, use a pedometer to track your mileage. Resembling a beeper that clips to your belt or waistband, a pedometer counts your steps during the day, or while you're doing your walking program. It is a great motivator that cues you to be more active. When you see or feel it on your waist, you're prompted to get moving. Use a pedometer to help yourself steadily increase the number of steps you walk each day. Increasing your steps translates into more calories burned.

- Try exercise poles. These are specially designed ski poles designed for use during walking. They stimulate the arm motion of cross-country skiing, thus boosting your upper body endurance and strengthening the arm and shoulder muscles used. Research shows you can burn roughly 20 percent more calories than someone walking the same pace without poles. They're great if you have knee or foot problems, too.

- Drink enough water. Before exercising, drink a cup of water. Continue to sip some water while exercising—about a half a cup or a full cup every 15 to 20 minutes. After exercising, replace any fluid you've lost by drinking an additional cup or two of water.

10

Key Seven:
Your Circle of Support
Unlock the Door to Social Control

*A friend is someone who walks in when others
walk out.*
—Walter Winchell

Key #7: Your circle of support.

Weight loss is not a do-it-yourself deal. If you expect to lose weight
and keep it off, you must build and nurture relationships that affirm
and uplift you in life-changing ways. Support from people you trust
will flow through you like a current, energizing you to get results and
have what you want. There is strength and power in support.

This key unlocks the door to *social control,* the ability to nurture
relationships built on trust, acceptance, and encouragement. It is
a fact of psychological functioning that when people attempt to
make lifestyle and behavioral changes, including diet and exercise
changes, they succeed over the long haul when they have genuinely
positive support provided by family, friends, coworkers, or from
professional sources such as physicians, therapists, ministers, or support groups. Thus, this key deals specifically with the people in your
life and the degree to which they support you or sabotage you. It
takes into account that the people around you aren't mind readers—
you have a responsibility to tell them what you want, what you expect, and what you're seeking so that you can tap into their support
to help you achieve your goals. With this key, I'll challenge you to
take step-through-door actions necessary to break free from entangle-

ments not in your best interest, and nurture a network of people who will support you in a meaningful, purposeful, and constructive manner.

Why is this key and its action-filled steps so important? Look at it this way: people will either contribute to or contaminate your personal weight control and management. Suppose, for example, that you came to see me because you wanted to lose 75 pounds. It might take several counseling sessions before you get on the right track because we would have to spend many hours talking about your lifestyle and your behavior. But suppose that I go to your house instead of you coming to see me. I meet your spouse and your mother-in-law, and they're both as wide as two axe handles. Bingo. I'm clued in right away: you're surrounded by other overweight people, and in all likelihood these relationships have influenced your weight in some monumentally negative ways.

Without question, your relationships powerfully impact your weight, your health, and your very well-being. They can influence the choices you make and affect your behavior, negatively and positively. With food, for example, we tend to eat more when we are in the company of others, and we tend to eat more of the wrong stuff. We tend to entertain ourselves with food if those in our social circle do the same. We might get suckered in to watching a football game all afternoon rather than going outside and playing a game of touch football. All of us are prone to doing what our family, friends, and close associates do, even if it is against our better judgment, because we want to fit in and be accepted. So we will generally conform to the behavior of the groups to which we belong. Our relationships have the fortunate or unfortunate tendency of pressuring us toward conformity. It's just the human way.

Sometimes this is healthy and constructive, while at other times it may be destructive. One of the dangers in conformity is expressed in the popular bumper sticker that says, "Don't follow me. I'm lost too." The wisdom of that bumper sticker should be clear. Watch out if you follow the crowd because they may not know where they're headed. There is a useful illustration here in drug addiction. If you have a problem with cocaine and you continue to hang out with other people who use cocaine, it is very likely that you will eventually use cocaine again. To live in a healthy manner, you've got to recognize the influence of your relationships on your life and take care that they don't push or pull you in the wrong direction.

SOCIAL SUPPORT AUDIT

How much support do you have in your life right now for what you are trying to accomplish? Take this quick true-false test designed to alert you to the levels of support or sabotage that currently exist in your relationships. Acknowledging these important aspects of your relational life can be liberating when you realize that at last you are getting real about what is going on. Circle true or false for all of the statements, whichever expresses exactly what is going on in your relationships. Again, don't be afraid to tell yourself the truth, even though it can be scary to admit certain things in your answers. The only thing worse about having nonsupportive relationships is to be in denial about those relationships. As is the case with any problem, early and appropriate intervention is vital to positive change.

My friends or family (whichever best applies):

1. Compliment me on healthy eating. **True/False**

2. Refuse to eat in a healthy manner. **True/False**

3. Notice when my behavior changes in significantly positive ways. **True/False**

4. Insist on taking me to fast-food restaurants and buffets. **True/False**

5. Compliment me on my appearance. **True/False**

6. Push foods that are a problem for me. **True/False**

7. Help me purchase and prepare healthy meals. **True/False**

8. Protest changes in the family diet. **True/False**

9. Help me overcome temptations to eat. **True/False**

10. Make fun of my efforts to lose weight. **True/False**

11. Offer to exercise with me. **True/False**

12. Complain about the time I spend exercising. **True/False**

13. Give me encouragement to exercise and stick with it. **True/False**

14. Buy and bring home low-response cost foods that are not good for me. **True/False**

15. Rearrange their schedules to exercise with me. **True/False**

16. Don't want me to exercise, or don't support my efforts. **True/False**

17. Talk to me about exercise in a positive manner. **True/False**

18. Schedule activities that interfere with my exercise time. **True/False**

19. Provide helpful information about nutrition, exercise, and health. **True/False**

20. Eat fattening foods in front of me. **True/False**

SCORING AND INTERPRETATION

Any odd-numbered questions to which you answered False, and even-numbered questions to which you answered True, score against your relationships in terms of the level of support provided by people in your life. You should look over your responses to get a feel for where support problems may exist. Don't get down on yourself or the people in your life, though. Being aware of these chinks in your relationships is a good thing, because I believe that you can deal with anything as long as you recognize it.

ACTION STEPS THROUGH THE DOOR TO SOCIAL CONTROL

Whenever you begin to take charge of your weight and your health, not all the people in your life will like it. In fact, some may belittle your efforts, they may make fun of you, they may tell you you can't do it, and they may urge you to eat food you don't need. You began to see this in the audit you just took. But these attitudes and behaviors don't mean that the people in your life are mean or evil; it's just that they don't want things to change. They have gotten comfortable with the deal the way it is, and they don't like it that you are changing the deal. People truly do fear change, especially if it affects their relationships and their lifestyle, and they will become frightened and will refuse to accept your changing the status quo. Maybe your husband worries that he will lose you to another man if you trim down. Maybe your best friend thinks you will get all the girls if you get in shape. Maybe your mom thinks you don't love her anymore if you refuse her fresh-baked apple pie for dessert every night. If the people closest to you get the idea that the "price of poker" is about to go way up, that you are going to stir up the norm all of sudden, they may feel threatened in a big way.

But no matter what the situation or motivation, if you allow yourself to be sidetracked by these reactions, you're in danger of veering off course—way, way off course. You must be very careful not to let others in your life deter you from your task of managing your weight. You can be sensitive to their fears and help them to a degree, but you must let them own and be responsible for their own feelings. This is about you, your weight, and your health; it is not about them.

Okay, let's move on to talking about your relationships and how they can work for you or against you specifically in terms of your weight management. To move closer to achieving your weight loss goals, it goes without saying that you need people in your life who will support you—friends, family members, and others who love you unconditionally and believe in you. By contrast, you must go on red-alert that there may be "saboteurs" in your life, some obvious, some not so obvious. These are people who will try to frustrate your efforts in various ways, and their behavior can obstruct your success if you're blind to their sabotage. The audit you just took hopefully provided a much-needed wake-up call to the degree of support or sabotage you have in your life at present.

In the action steps that follow, you'll find instructions on what to do with those who would sabotage you, intentionally or unintentionally, and how to inoculate yourself against their manipulation. Because your circle of support is so critical to your success, we'll also talk about how to choose the right team to help you do what you have to do, as you make critical changes in your lifestyle. Here's a point-by-point look at how to build genuine support in your life.

STEP ONE: SORT OUT THE SABOTEURS FROM THE SUPPORTERS

In working with overweight clients, I have observed the dynamics of people who react toxically to your desire to lose weight and get in shape. You need to know these dynamics so that you won't be sabotaged along the way to your desired weight.

Saboteurs can be obstacles in your path to weight loss. Be on the alert for these saboteurs and their behavior patterns. Be cautious when you are the most vulnerable, and always have a plan in place for dealing with them. They are not directly trying to harm your weight loss efforts; rather they are trying to protect their own lives and interests. They are getting in your way because you have gotten in their way, by changing how you eat, changing your looks, or changing a style of living that has become familiar and comfortable to them. If you can spot their sabotage, how you handle them depends on which type of saboteur you're at odds with. There are four types of saboteurs whom I typically see as being among the most likely to try, on purpose or not, to thwart your efforts toward your goal.

The Food Pusher

This type of saboteur is among the most common: your mother who lovingly but relentlessly pushes her homemade brownies at you, even though she knows you're trying to lose weight; the party hostess who says "You can go off your diet just this once," enticing you with second helpings of mashed potatoes and gravy; your coworker who says at coffee breaks, "You've just got to try my homemade cinnamon rolls"; or even your spouse, who brings chocolate-covered cherries home to you once too often.

Food pushers like these can be extremely undermining because their methods are virtually invisible. They seem so loving, so well-intentioned. Their influence, however subtle, can be especially powerful because it typically comes from people you trust—your parents, grandparents, relatives, spouse, and close friends. The food they want you to eat is offered in the name of love and concern, making it very hard to resist, particularly if you don't want to hurt their feelings.

Understand that food pushers may be attempting to seek approval from you, and in doing so, are trying to manipulate you into eating food to please themselves. They may have an insatiable appetite for reassurance and stroking, and one way they attempt to get it is to constantly fish for compliments about their cooking. They may not believe in themselves enough, and so they look for a higher degree of self-worth in externals, either people or circumstances.

Many times, a Food Pusher—especially if she's your mother or grandmother—simply does not know how to support you as an adult and is more comfortable treating you as child who must be fed and nourished. She is used to loving you with food; it's the only way she knows. By refusing her food, you're saying you don't want to be loved that way anymore. She winds up feeling hurt and rejected.

It's important for you to recognize these behaviors in people with whom you share your life, but at the same time, you must steel yourself against their persuasiveness. Be kind when you can, but firm when you must. You alone are responsible for what you put in your mouth, and what you do to get in shape. If the people in your life don't get this, then that's their problem, not yours.

The Control Freak

With the Control Freak, it's all about power manipulation. The Control Freak is dead set on sabotaging your personal control and power over your ability to manage your weight. I vividly recall a couple I worked with for several months who were seriously considering divorce rather than continuing their hostile marriage. Darren and Sara had been married barely two years. For Sara, it was her first marriage; for Darren, his second. Years earlier, Darren's first wife had had an affair, and one day Darren came home to a house stripped bare of all their possessions. His wife left him for the other guy, and divorce soon followed. Though deeply wounded and dazed by the rejection, Darren attempted to get on with his life. A friend introduced him to Sara on a blind date, and a whirlwind courtship ensued. Sara was attractive, bubbly, and smart, but in sharp contrast to his first wife, about 30 pounds overweight. The weight, however, was not a sexual turnoff for Darren. After nine months of dating, Darren and Sara tied the knot.

Shortly after getting married, Sara decided to diet and exercise at a local gym in order to lose weight. Darren began to grow uneasy. At first, he started picking at Sara, complaining that she was leaving the house too often to go to exercise classes instead of spending time with him. He began to criticize the meals she cooked and griped that they tasted too bland, like Styrofoam. In attempts to get his way, Darren would spout guilt-inducing phrases like, "If you loved me, you'd cook food I like. If you really cared about me, you'd stop spending all that time at the gym." The only kind words he ever spoke seemed to be, "I like you fat."

This behavior began to escalate. Darren forbade Sara to go to exercise classes, and he even forbade her to wear makeup. He began bringing home all sorts of fattening foods, including candy, cakes, bakery breads, and so forth. In retaliation, Sara lashed out with in-your-face obscenities and other verbal poison. The only way she could calm down after these venomous arguments was to binge on ungodly amounts of sugary, high-fat foods. There was no way she could lose weight in the midst of this mental and emotional turmoil. The viciousness on both sides had torn them apart, and the relationship was going down in flames.

In therapy, as our interactions wore on, it was apparent that Darren was terribly insecure personally. He was so afraid that Sara would leave him as his first wife had, that he did everything he could to control her appearance. The fatter and more unattractive she stayed, according to Darren's sick reasoning, the less likely she was to stray. He had a pathological fear that he'd lose Sara to another man if she lost weight, so he felt he had to keep her fat. He'd rather have her fat than not have her at all.

Obviously, there were a lot of complex issues to work on. Darren had to make a decision about whether he wanted to persist in his control-freak role, allowing it to dominate his every waking hour, or get real and take the risk of letting himself love and trust. It was clear to me that if he didn't, Sara would be out of there—and not for the reasons Darren feared most.

Ultimately, this couple did decide to examine their behaviors with a very critical eye so as to stop the sabotage, both of their marriage and of Sara's desire to get in shape. By confronting their shortcomings and resolving these control issues, Darren and Sara did eventually save their marriage. Darren was transformed from a saboteur into a supporter, once he realized how much he was hurting Sara and the relationship. Sara, in turn, learned to stop her attack-dog behavior by focusing and building on the admirable qualities that had originally attracted her to Darren. Working through their problems strengthened the bonds between them, and today they plan healthy meals together and serve as each other's training partners in their gym. Sara, by the way, is another success story, weighing a healthy 125 pounds, thanks to Darren's loving support and the transformation in their relationship.

Learn to evaluate the messages you receive from those closest to you. Is your mate telling you that you can't because he or she will feel threatened if you do? Is your friend or relative acting out of fear? Remember what I said earlier: people who genuinely care about you still get really scared when you try to change. In response, they'll try to keep you protectively wrapped up in their cocoon so that you'll yield to the authority of their power.

If there's a Control Freak in your life right now, be forthright. You may have to reassure him or her that yes, things are changing, but this does not mean that your friendship, affection, or love will change. Your overall attitude about what you're trying to accomplish should allow for no second-guessing on the part of people in your life.

The Green-Eyed Monster

Think about some of your friends who might be too unmotivated to address their own weight problems or start an exercise program. Then you show up on the scene, looking lighter and more in shape than the last time they saw you.

Jealousy, envy, and resentment erupt with all the force of a long-dormant volcano.

Sure, they might hover over you with words like, "You look great . . . how'd you do it?" while inwardly they're thinking, "That bitch!"

These people—the Green-Eyed Monsters of the saboteurs—are not really happy over your success. They're just plain jealous that you're looking so good, and they'll try to control you with their jealousy and sabotage your efforts. This may take the form of words like "You're losing too much weight," or "You look too thin," or "Don't you think you're taking this diet thing too seriously?" Be on guard for such comments, since they're not made out of sincere regard for your health, but rather out of envy. Be aware too, that their behavior may manifest itself in actions like pushing food. Whatever the behavior, the Green-Eyed Monsters will try to get you off your program and bring you down to their fitness level or to a fitness level lower than the one they themselves occupy. Even though they'd hate to admit it, they'd love nothing more than to see you fail, or get in worse shape than they're in.

Keep in mind that often, Green-Eyed Monsters are the same people who are too afraid to confront badly needed lifestyle changes in their own lives. They're only getting on your case because they haven't been able to do anything about their own. They feel guilty because they haven't been successful at taking charge of their own physical health.

Tell the Green-Eyed Monster that his or her behavior is putting up a brick wall between the two of you. Unless that wall comes tumbling down, the sense of trust and honest communication that once existed between you will be lost.

Don't be deterred from achieving your weight loss goals just because somebody else is too afraid or unmotivated to go after their own. Remember that it's not somebody else's responsibility to tell you what you should eat, or how much you should weigh. You alone are responsible for your weight and your health. What's more, no one has the power to persuade you to abandon your goals unless you let them.

The Statue

There may be people in your life who will not encourage you to change because they want—consciously or otherwise—to maintain the status quo. I call these saboteurs the Statues because they turn rigid and inflexible whenever you want to make positive lifestyle changes. They prefer the status quo because it is a safe, comfortable place to be. If you're the family cook, for example, and you've decided that everyone is going to eat healthier meals, it won't be long before your family hatches a conspiracy to "get Mom off her diet." If you've stopped drinking beer with your buddies on Friday night, expect them to resent it. They'll hate that the phrase "six-pack" now accurately describes your abs, not your drinking capacity—so be prepared for them to try to drag you back down to their level for the sake of their own comfort.

It's just that once you decide to make a change, some of the people in your life will resist that change. This shift of position by you is seen as a major threat to all. Your decision may trigger resistance: the saboteur may rise up against the perceived threat. You may get messages like, "You're no fun anymore," or "Aren't we ever going to go out to eat again?"

Winning support from Statues is tough, particularly if you've tried to lose weight in the past but have failed. Every attempt on your part looks so unstable, and they count on you to fail. They may even remind you: "Why even try? Look what happened the last time you did this."

As with any sabotage, this type of pressure can make you less likely to stick to the changes you want to make. The key is to never let anyone take your commitment away from you, especially not for the sake of their own comfort.

Do This Exercise

Are there saboteurs in your life? If so, it's critical to know how to deal with them. In this exercise, I'd like you to write down the names of people you feel might sabotage your weight loss efforts, intentionally or unintentionally. Look back at the four descriptions of saboteurs I've given you, and next to each name, write down the category of sabotage that fits (some people may fit more than one category). Please understand that this is not a faultfinding exercise. It's just a way to scan your personal radar screen for the people who might derail your weight-management efforts even in the kindest of well-intended ways.

Next, decide upon the response you might give. Are you going to avoid the person altogether? Will you sit down with them and explain the program you're on, and why, so that they understand your motivations? Will you let them know that their negative attitude or behavior is destructive and that it's interfering with your chance to lose weight? If it's a relationship partner who feels threatened, will you tell him or her that even though you're changing your lifestyle, your love will stay the same? Will you simply figure out some gracious ways of saying "no" when food is pushed your way? Let the chart below guide your planning.

CHART 3. HOW I WILL DEAL WITH SABOTEURS

DEALING WITH SABOTEURS		
Possible Saboteur	*Type of Saboteur*	*My Response*

Please remember that most people whom you love and respect are not people who want to harm you and your health. I'm sure that these are wonderful people, but this does not mean that they always know what is in your best interests. Friends and family do not always plan to get you off your program. Some do it out of a desire to mother you. Others are trying to protect a relationship, or protect themselves from change. Still others may be trying to protect the predictable world that the two of you share.

Even so, I have to be honest with you here: it is difficult to fight your weight battles if you have to fight your friends and family at the same time. You need people to believe in you, and if they cannot do that, then you may also need to re-invent your relationships and surround yourself with people who will. It is your right to choose those people who will be around you while you work on your weight and your health; you have this right and you must claim it unapologetically. Don't continue to pretend that you don't know who has your best interests at heart and who does not. You know it as surely as you are sitting there. Give yourself permission to act on that knowledge and claim your right to a healthy existence. Once you do so, you will see the world start standing up and taking notice.

Bottom line: surround yourself with people who will move in the direction of your goals. Read on, and you'll find out how to build a team of people who can help you function at your best.

STEP TWO: ASSEMBLE YOUR SUPPORTING TEAM

Considering that there may be saboteurs in your vicinity, you must make a conscious effort to recruit the supporting team that you need. Having designed life strategies for so many people just like you, I've observed that you can build support in highly effective ways—if you add to your support-building an element of fun and creativity.

Lyle's story is typical of what I am talking about, and although it involves smoking cessation, it applies universally to any situation in which you need support for a lifestyle change. At work, Lyle would habitually purchase cigarettes from a vending machine, and this habit had become a real blockade to his quitting. At my suggestion, he printed out a stack of cards to distribute to his coworkers. On those cards were the following instructions: *Please do not give me a cigarette and please do not give me money to buy cigarettes. I am trying to quit smoking and I need your support.* When it became clear to his coworkers that Lyle was serious, but that he was approaching it in an amusing, nonthreatening way, they responded supportively. Just like Lyle, you must remain resolute in your determination but at the same time try humor, fun, and creativity to melt the resistance of those who may not yet be cheering you on.

In assembling your supporters, you must decide who will be on your team and who will not, who will be a part of your support circle, and whom you need to be with you. You have the right to choose your own team, and if you want to succeed, you will go about this with care and deliberation. To guide you in your thinking, let me introduce you to four "team members" who can be indispensable and invaluable as you go forward.

The Coach

The Coach is someone with technical expertise or professional training who can provide knowledge on nutrition, exercise, or some other aspect of health management. Personal trainers, exercise instructors, support group facilitators, nutritionists, therapists, and physicians are examples of people who may serve as coaches in your life. They have the information, the resources, the guidance, the insight, and the answers to your questions. These are people who provide practical help and have the background and education to do so. Their motivating power lies partially in their status as authority figures; it is a well-known premise of social psychology that authority figures do have a huge impact on behavior. A Coach can be a genuinely positive influence in your life, particularly if you are just learning the ropes of exercising and eating right. Counsel from the Coach opens up opportunities and new ways to do things that you didn't know existed, or unravels for you a problem you thought had no solution. Often, a Coach is a role model, living in a healthy way that challenges you to live your life with the same positive qualities you appreciate and admire.

The Teammate

As you assemble your support circle, you may want to team up with someone—a Teammate—whose weight loss and fitness goals are similar to your own. Your Teammate could be your spouse or a close friend, a companion with whom you share a sense of purpose that keeps you both on task. This is someone with whom you work out, someone who's following the same program you're on, someone who helps you prepare healthy food, or someone who joins you on recreational outings. You and your Teammate can help monitor each other's behavior, comparing notes on what's working and what's not, and rallying to each other's aid if needed. Teammates can play a unique and substantial role in your life because they are natural motivators. After all, you're less likely to duck out on your exercise session if your Teammate is counting on you to be there. In recruiting a Teammate, find someone with a passion that is contagious. Whenever you are around your Teammate, you will begin to share in his or her excitement and purpose. You will be energized and impassioned, and your healthiest behaviors will be strengthened.

The Cheerleader

The Cheerleader gives you honest, meaningful words of encouragement, building you up at critical times and offering support without a hint of judgmental attitude. What the Cheerleader is not is a person who tells you you're doing great even though you've eaten a half-dozen doughnuts every day for breakfast. Whoever this person might be, he or she has an affirming presence in your life, in a caring and responsible way. The Cheerleader is someone who causes you to believe that your goals are something worth having, and steers you gently toward achieving those goals. I recall one patient telling me, for example, that his wife "tricked him into working out," by encouraging him to walk to a nearby book store several times a week for coffee. Initially, he hated exercise and was so out of shape that it was physically taxing just to get a few steps out the door. But he kept at it and is now a confirmed jogger who dropped several trouser sizes because of his wife's gentle cheerleading. Knowing that your Cheerleader is there to support you from a heart level, brings energy and strength to your efforts in immeasurable ways. Every one needs a Cheerleader or two, because the Cheerleader can be your greatest fan.

The Umpire

With a candor and honesty that is refreshing, the Umpire is someone who's ready to give you constructive feedback and inspiring responses. This is someone who cares about you enough to tell you the truth, constructively and helpfully. What distinguishes the Umpire is that he or she is a good listener and observer—someone alert, interested, responsive, and never distracted when engaged in meaningful conversation with you. There is such a high level of trust in this relationship that you're able to share your feelings and reveal where you're vulnerable. Upbeat and empathetic, the Umpire listens carefully to you in order to determine the appropriate response or course of action. More often than not, this is to help you think through problems so that you come up with your own answers. This kind of relationship always increases your chance for success, because the Umpire stands by you no matter how deep your personal conflict or distress.

An important caveat here is that the people in your circle of support may not all fit neatly into the Coach, Teammate, Cheerleader, or Umpire categories. Some of your supporters may have all four characteristics, admirable and motivating in all kinds of ways. If you have such a person or circle of people, then you are indeed blessed—and you should continue to nurture these relationships even after you have lost your weight and have it under control. These are people who have had a hand in your success. Keeping them in your life is critical to your long-term health and happiness.

If, for whatever reason, the people close to you are still reluctant in their support, sometimes you have to send them an ultimatum that states who will be a member of your team and who will not. Be considerate, but firm; don't stop short of telling them what you want and what you need. Some of the people in your immediate circle are simply not going to change their sabotaging spirit, but you can certainly change your reaction to them. Think about it: you can seldom change those in your life. But what you can change is the manner in which you engage them. The first person that you need to assert yourself with is you. When you move your position on yourself, when you stand up for yourself and for your right to have what you want, you may find that people in your life stop sabotaging you because you've taught them that they can't.

It is a hard but true reality that you may even have to get some new friends, at least during the time you're at work on your task. You must decide that you would rather be healthy by yourself than be fat with other people. This shows you are not bluffing, you are not blowing hot and cold, and you are in the game to the last. It means that you would rather be by yourself, treating yourself with dignity and respect and living healthfully and happily, than be around people you cannot count on. You may have a habit of being with certain people, but if they are disinclined to treat you reasonably and properly, and jeopardize your health, then maybe it's time for you to part company in order to do what you have to do.

STEP THREE: REOPEN THE NEGOTIATIONS WITH YOUR FAMILY

As for your immediate family, don't think for a second that I am suggesting that you ditch a spouse or kids who incline toward being non-supportive. What I am suggesting is that you reopen the negotiations on how your family should function. Look at it this way: you taught your family the rules, you fried the chicken, you baked the cookies, you drove them to McDonald's, and they, like you, have gotten accustomed to the same-old, same-old way of living. But if that way of living is about to take a sharp turn, then it's only fair that you prepare them for what's around the corner. If you have taught someone how to play a certain game, then change the rules, the rest of the players are entitled to know the new rules.

As you reopen the negotiations, you must commit to do so from a position of strength and resolve, not from insecurity and self-doubt. The worst thing you could do is make a lot of noise about changing your lifestyle, only to revert to the old, familiar, destructive patterns. To talk about change and not do it is to teach your family to discount your declarations and commitments as empty, meaningless words. Stay the course. You might begin your renegotiation conversations with words like these:

I need your loving support and cooperation.

Please give me encouragement.

Help me do this with your praise and compliments.

Bring me nonfood gifts and rewards like flowers, books, music, or pampering at a salon.

Give me affection, but not expressed with food.

I'd love it if you'd offer me healthy food.

Let's rearrange our schedule so we can exercise together or do something fun and recreational.

Let me explain the keys I'm using and the steps I'm taking toward achieving my weight loss goals.

Would you like to try to eat the same healthy foods I'm eating?

Let's discuss my progress and minimize our conversations about food.

Be a partner in my program. My success is your success.

Lift me up when I'm tempted and about to fall.

Do not waffle and do not be dissuaded from your resolve. Where your well-being is concerned, commit to yourself that, although it may be difficult to effect change in your relationships, you must not compromise. To compromise in this area is to sell out your dreams and goals of losing weight and having a healthier, more satisfying life.

STEP FOUR: CREATE ACCOUNTABILITY

Reporting your progress to an external accountability source—someone in your trusted circle of family and friends—has enormous motivating value and is an important part of goal setting, as I pointed out

244 / THE ULTIMATE WEIGHT SOLUTION

in Chapter 2. I promise you, you will respond better if you know that somebody is checking up on you. This approach has been used successfully with groups such as Alcoholics Anonymous (AA) in which recovering alcoholics are assigned a "sponsor" to help them stay sober.

Another way to create accountability is to join a support group for people like you who have weight and overeating problems. These groups are helpful if you ever come to feel that the people in your life do not understand your challenges, what you are going through, and how you feel. As a member of a support group, you can meet others who are working on the same problems and with whom you can share your victories and your struggles. Ultimately, you must work on your weight problem yourself—you are accountable first to yourself—but you can tap into the resources of a group for mutual support and accountability. But make sure the support group you join has a focus toward the positive, in which its members share what is working for them without whining, without complaints, and without excuses. If there is a spirit of negativity in the air, this can drain the joy and encouragement from the experience. When you leave a support group each time, you should feel encouraged, inspired, and uplifted. If, on the other hand, you feel down and discouraged then that's not the group for you, and you should discontinue your participation.

Without accountability, you are apt to let yourself off the hook, failing to recognize slipping behavior in time to adjust and keep from falling short. So go public with someone you trust, and find support when you need it. This will be a person, or a group, to whom you make periodic reports on your progress. In doing so, you would have step-by-step accountability, perhaps reporting to your accountability source every Friday afternoon to review how many pounds you lost that week, the frequency and duration of your weekly exercise sessions, or even your failure to accomplish what's required. Faced with this level of accountability, you are now motivated to stay on track, since you will be scrutinized on a weekly basis.

Some days you might feel like eating right and exercising; some days you might not. But if you know precisely what you want, how to get there, and the time and places are scheduled and time-protected, and there are real consequences for falling short, you are much more likely to continue in your pursuit of your goal.

So set up an accountability source for yourself who will make it impossible for you not to achieve your goals. Always remember that it is your job to manage your weight; it is your accountability source's job to help and support you. Ultimately, only you—and you alone—are responsible for getting your weight under control.

As you use this key, please don't be a lone ranger. If you're isolated, you'll have a tougher time keeping your weight down. Gather around yourself a cadre of people with whom you can healthfully interact—people who care about you and have your best interests at heart. What matters is that you have people in your life who want you to succeed, not just for today, next week, or next month, but for the rest of your life. This is a supremely important key to permanent weight loss and control.

Part Three

POWERFUL INSIGHTS

11

When You Can't
Lose Weight
Are You Weight Loss Resistant?

Don't compromise yourself. You are all you've got.
—BETTY FORD

For many of you, weight control has been an elusive, self-punishing struggle for which there seems to be no answer. No matter what you do, the pounds won't budge. Although the usual suspects in weight gain are poor choices, bad habits, wrong thinking, emotional over-eating, and so forth, there are certain underlying medical issues that can pack on weight. If this situation is happening to you, it is no small injustice, but please be encouraged that medical conditions contributing to weight gain are known and correctable. The reason I am so confident about this is because a couple of years ago, I found myself in a similar predicament—I was having to work much too hard to maintain what was for me a very stable weight, a weight that felt good and natural.

There were subtle but undeniable tip-offs that something was wrong. Some afternoons during my usual game of tennis, I felt heavy, as though I were slogging around in slow-motion, and I was getting tired much too easily.

Having been a jock practically all of my life, I stay in reasonably good shape, with a definite impetus for doing so. As I told you in the beginning of the book, I grew up in a family with a long history of obesity, which sadly has been an instigator of serious health problems in my immediate family. I give credit to a lifetime in athletics—my earlier years in football and more recently on the tennis court—for sparing me from obesity. To this day, I exercise aerobically and lift weights, at a high level of discipline and intensity, because I firmly believe that maximum performance requires a work-your-butt-off commitment. And as someone who consistently makes good nutritional choices, I can honestly say that I eat more vegetables and other healthy stuff than Quaker has oats.

But at age fifty-one, I was fighting way, way too hard to hold onto my target weight. Following the only logic I knew, I responded by requiring even more of myself—more exercise, and stricter monitoring of my food intake, as to both quality and quantity. With everything I was doing, I should have been as thin as a gnat's whisker. But believe me, it was like running uphill in foot-deep mud to even stay close to holding my own! Prior formulas for success, as well as everything I knew should be working, were not working at all.

I knew that there was a problem; I just didn't know what was causing this newfound resistance, especially since I was no "Johnny-come-lately." I had spent a lifetime as an athlete, yet I was losing ground. And I subscribe to the strategy that if what you're doing isn't working, do something different. So I did.

I underwent a thorough physical, including a series of laboratory tests, to decipher whether there was anything amiss in my body chemistry, the reactionary stew of substances in the body, from hormones to blood sugar to blood fats, that figure into metabolism.

Soon afterwards, my doctor called with the results and dropped the bombshell. My triglycerides (components of fat that float around in the blood) were dangerously elevated. My blood sugar was soaring on the high side of normal, indicating that my body was not processing sugar well and a lot of it was being converted into sustainable body fat. I was blown away by the revelations that emerged from this testing, but fortunately both conditions were correctable through proper nutritional and medical management.

Knowing this was a huge relief—huge. But the information also foretold something more threatening: that unless I got my triglycerides and blood sugar under control, I was galloping toward heart disease or diabetes. Truthfully, the imbalances might not affect me for another five or ten years or so—nothing had really broken down yet—but I knew that the consequences would be very real at some point in my life. The results of my tests were a shrill wake-up call. My body was telling me through these metabolic problems that I was on the road to some very serious diseases. Now that I knew, I was sure listening.

What ultimately turned the corner for me was a prescribed regimen of nutritional supplements, diet, and medication to rebalance my body chemistry and get me aligned medically. Each of these measures worked dramatically; my weight dropped back down to a normal, comfortable range and has stayed there ever since.

Question: is it possible that, just like me, you could have something going on inside your body that is preventing you from losing the weight you want to lose?

Absolutely. Of the 65 percent of our population that is overweight, there is a group of people who are what I term "weight loss resistant," with an inability to lose weight, even on effective weight loss and exercise programs, because of problems with individual biochemistry and metabolism.

You may be among these people who are hopelessly overweight with no idea as to why. If so, it may mean that you are biochemically and metabolically configured in such a way that you cannot lose a reasonable amount of weight and you cannot get results—no matter how disciplined you are, no matter how much you sacrifice, and no matter how much get-trim torture you put yourself through. You can go on the same diet, the same exercise program, and the same self-improvement stuff as your best friend, but when it's all said and done, your butt will still be as big as two hams in a tow sack, and she'll be so skinny that her body doesn't look lived in. Bottom line: it's alarmingly easy for you to put on pounds and alarmingly difficult for you to take them off.

If you are living with obesity that you neither caused nor wanted, the problems could be in your own physiology, not necessarily in your diet or in your lifestyle. Your body may be playing a nasty trick on you, and as a result, your excessive weight seems to be an unavoidable destiny. Yes, it's a raw deal, but it is not a sealed fate. You can outsmart your body with the right medical treatment and intervention.

No matter how frustrated you may feel right now, please don't tune me out. I am one of the very few people who knows exactly what you've been through; I lived it in my own life. I know what it's like when eating right and exercising hard don't go your way. So if you're tired of being stuck, then you've come to the right place. Together, we are going to get you out of this trap and make your weight manageable again.

ARE YOU WEIGHT LOSS RESISTANT?

Dieting and exercising if you are weight loss resistant is like trying to drown, trap, or poison the moles ruining your beautifully manicured lawn. Those things will not work alone, because you are attacking the wrong problem. The real problem is the grubs in the ground the moles are feeding on. Exterminate the grubs, and you get rid of the moles.

So before you can get rid of the fat that's glued to your hips or circling your stomach, you've got to find out what's making you weight loss resistant. This is a crucial question that must be answered up front. Unless you get to the heart of it, you won't lose much weight at all, no matter what you do, and your own body will continue to sabotage you from the inside out. You cannot change what you don't acknowledge. You can't be sure if you don't ask.

Let's begin to find out, with a simple profile to determine the possibility that you may indeed be weight loss resistant. This profile is not meant to take the place of a thorough medical checkup by your physician; it should be used only as a first step toward identifying weight loss resistance.

Take the time to answer each question as honestly as you can. Don't cop out and say "yes, that's me" to every question, when in reality you are covering up for all those second helpings you've obviously helped yourself to. Too many "yes" responses may mean that you are trying to hunt for excuses for being overweight, that you would rather pin your weight problem elsewhere because you do not have the conscious resolve to change your lifestyle and behavior. So please—be honest when you answer these questions. Unless you are, you will misidentify and ultimately mistreat your problem, never truly fixing it. You will neglect what needs medical attention.

WEIGHT LOSS RESISTANCE PROFILE

In the following profile, you will see that the numbered questions ask you to answer "yes" or "no." Next to each question, circle the answer that best describes your personal situation. If you are unsure about your answer, leave it blank, but try to answer all seven questions as accurately and as honestly as you can.

1. Are you unable to lose weight despite repeated dieting attempts and a regular exercise program? **Yes/No**

2. Are you taking one or more of the following medications: hormone replacement therapy (HRT), antidepressants (specifically a class of drugs known as "SSRIs" or tricyclic antidepressants), diabetic medications, steroids, blood pressure drugs, or antiseizure medications? **Yes/No**

3. Have you recently experienced two or more of the following symptoms: intolerance to cold and changes in temperature; fatigue; constipation; skin that is dry, coarse, or pale; hoarseness in your voice; thinning hair; poor memory; difficulty concentrating? **Yes/No**

4. Measure your waist with a tape measure positioned one inch above your navel. Is your waist measurement greater than 35 inches if you are a woman or greater than 40 inches if you are a man? **Yes/No**

5. At your last annual physical, were you told by your doctor that you have three or more of the following conditions: high blood pressure, elevated triglycerides (150 or higher), low HDL cholesterol (less than 50), or elevated blood sugar? **Yes/No**

6. Do you tend to gain weight primarily around your hips and thighs? **Yes/No**

7. (Women only) Have you recently experienced two or more of the following symptoms: mood changes, tender breasts, menstrual (bleeding) changes, dryness in genitals, hot flashes, or excessive sweating? **Yes/No**

SCORING AND INTERPRETATION

If you truthfully answered "yes" to two or more of these questions, this quite possibly indicates that you are weight loss resistant. In reality, there is only one way to find out for sure, and that is through extensive medical assessment and testing. Please read on.

HOW TO TELL IF YOU'RE WEIGHT LOSS RESISTANT: MEDICAL TESTING

As I did, the most important move to make is to seek medical testing and advice. Tell your doctor that you cannot lose weight, especially if you have been gaining weight, or have not been able to lose weight despite a focused program of diet and exercise. You may want to share with your doctor the results of the profile you just took. Your doctor may have greater knowledge about your condition, but you have greater knowledge about yourself, how you feel, and what you sense in your own body. It is your responsibility to supply the evidence that will steer your doctor in the right direction. Most of the time, an accurate description of your symptoms will lead your doctor to a more accurate diagnosis.

If your doctor is thorough and methodical, he or she will ask you key questions about your health when assessing you for medical problems. One of these questions may focus on the medications you're taking. Surprisingly, there are more than one hundred prescription medicines with the common side effect of weight gain, and you may be on one or more of them right now. Some of the biggest culprits are some common antidepressants, high blood pressure drugs, steroids, diabetic medications, hormone replacement therapy (HRT), and antiseizure medications. Note whether you are taking any of these so you can discuss your medication regimen with your physician. In fact, bring your doctor a list of all the prescribed and nonprescribed medications you are taking, and discuss it with your doctor. But very important: never discontinue taking any medication without first consulting your physician.

If medications are ruled out, chances are there may be a hormonal or metabolic problem. In the section that follows, I will briefly describe these conditions, along with the required diagnostic tests and how to interpret the results of those tests in light of your inability to lose weight.

UNDERACTIVE THYROID

Many people who struggle without success to lose weight are suffering from an underactive thyroid, in which the production of thyroid hormones slows or stops altogether. When this happens, your metabolism slows to a crawl too, and your body begins to store more calories as fat. Symptoms of an underactive thyroid include: intolerance to cold and temperature changes, fatigue, constipation, changes in your skin texture (increased paleness, coarseness, or dryness), hoarseness in your voice, thinning hair, and memory problems. If your doctor suspects an underactive thyroid, *thyroid function tests* will be ordered and analyzed. These tests check your blood for levels of thyroid hormones, known medically as TSH, Free T3, and Free T4.

Once you and your doctor have the results of your thyroid function tests in hand, there are questions you should ask in order to find out how your thyroid function is blocking your efforts to lose weight. The accompanying table will help you interpret your results, and provides guidance on what to ask your doctor about your tests results. If you have an underactive thyroid, it is treated and corrected with supplemental thyroid medication, taken daily for life.

METABOLIC SYNDROME

Involving mostly problems with blood sugar and blood fats, Metabolic Syndrome is a cluster of disorders that together may be causing your body to convert too many calories into fat. Truthfully, overeating and getting too little exercise are the main instigators of this syndrome. And once you've got it, you're staring down the barrel of a real dilemma. Metabolic Syndrome sets you up for heart attack, stroke, full-blown type II diabetes, certain cancers, and liver disease. Because your blood chemistry and metabolism are negatively affected, losing weight becomes all the more challenging. But that's what you've got to do—shed your excess pounds and become more active—in order to treat and overcome Metabolic Syndrome. In fact, dropping just 5 to

TABLE 9. THYROID FUNCTION TESTS: RESULTS AND INTERPRETATION

THYROID FUNCTION TESTS	*WHAT DO MY RESULTS MEAN?	HOW DO MY LAB RESULTS AFFECT MY WEIGHT?
TSH	Normal: 0.5 to 5.5 Optimal: 1 to 4 Abnormal: Technically, abnormal is greater than 5.5, but you may have difficulty losing weight with levels above 5.	This is considered to be the most sensitive test for your thyroid. An *elevated* TSH means that your body needs more thyroid activity. Specifically, a reading of between 4 and 5 may suggest that TSH is trying to get your thyroid to increase its production of the thyroid hormones, T3 and T4. Obviously, this isn't happening, and your body's ability to burn calories has slowed down. It's difficult to lose weight under these circumstances.
Free T3 and Free T4	Values vary greatly between labs; however, any decreased level needs to be addressed.	Decreased levels mean that your metabolism is sluggish. Consequently, you're not burning up enough energy, and your attempts at weight loss will remain in gridlock until your doctor initiates treatment and you comply with it.

* Values may vary depending upon laboratory used and your age and gender.

10 percent of your weight will greatly improve your body's handling of blood sugar and enhance your metabolism for the better.

The principal components of Metabolic Syndrome include abdominal obesity, elevated or high normal blood sugar, low blood levels of the "healthy" cholesterol (HDL), high blood levels of triglycerides, and high blood pressure. There is not one single test that should be performed, but rather a series of tests, for your doctor to make an accurate diagnosis. Most of these tests are performed routinely, usually as part of your annual medical checkup.

The table below lists the tests you should request, what the results of those tests might be, and how to interpret these results in light of weight loss resistance. Abnormalities here are typically treated with diet, supplements, and corrective doses of prescription medications. (For more information on treatment strategies, refer to the section entitled Overcoming Weight Loss Resistance found in this chapter, beginning on page 260.)

TABLE 10. METABOLIC SYNDROME TESTS: RESULTS AND INTERPRETATION

METABOLIC TESTS	*WHAT DO MY RESULTS MEAN?	HOW DO MY LAB RESULTS AFFECT MY WEIGHT?
Waist Circumference	Abnormal (women): Greater than 35 inches Abnormal (men): Greater than 40 inches	A waist circumference that exceeds normal is an important visual indicator of weight loss resistance.
Fasting Blood Glucose	Optimal: 80 Normal: Less than 110 Abnormal: Greater than 110 Risky: Greater than 126 (this indicates that you are at risk for diabetes)	If your fasting level falls in the upper range of 100 to 109, this means that you are starting to lose control of your blood sugar. Specifically, your body may be processing excess carbohydrates into fat, making it difficult for you to lose weight.
Triglycerides	Normal: Less than 150 Borderline-high: 150 to 199 High: 200 to 499 Very high: 500 or greater	Any value above 150 may indicate that your body is converting too much carbohydrate into triglycerides, which in turn can lead to fat gain.
HDL Cholesterol	Low: Less than 40 High: Greater than 60	Low HDL cholesterol puts you at high risk for heart disease. It may also point to an excess of refined carbohydrates and saturated fats in your diet. A reading of less than 40 in men and less than 50 in women is common in Metabolic Syndrome. The higher the HDL, the better. Remember, the H in HDL stands for healthy.

(continued on next page)

METABOLIC TESTS	*WHAT DO MY RESULTS MEAN?	HOW DO MY LAB RESULTS AFFECT MY WEIGHT?
Triglycerides/ HDL Ratio	Normal Ratio: Less than 4.5 Abnormal Ratio: Above 4.5 range	If your ratio falls in the 4 to 4.5 range, keep your eye on this number. It's a red flag, signaling poor blood sugar control and a tendency for your body to pack away excess carbohydrates as fat.
Blood Pressure	Normal: 120/80 Prehypertensive: Between 120/80 to 139/89 High: 140/90 or greater	A reading of 130/85 or greater is a risk factor for Metabolic Syndrome and the weight loss resistance that frequently accompanies it.

* *As a general medical rule, you will be diagnosed with Metabolic Syndrome when three or more abnormal conditions are present.*

ESTROGEN IMBALANCE

Another possibility, if you are a woman, is to look at your estrogen levels. Over your lifetime, if you have taken birth control pills, hormone replacement therapy (HRT), or both, your body may have built up an unhealthy surplus of estrogen, and one unfortunate outcome is that you are now packing fat on your thighs, hips, and rear. Other symptoms include mood changes, tender breasts, menstrual (bleeding) changes, dryness in genitals, and hot flashes or excessive sweating.

Doctors can test for estrogen imbalances with urine tests as well as with blood tests, although urine tests are more common. Normal values, based on your life stage, appear in Table 11 and will help you understand the meaning of your results, as well as what to ask your doctor. If your number is higher than the top number in each of these ranges, there is a strong probability that you have estrogen imbalance. If weight loss resistance is associated with estrogen problems, then either an adjustment or outright discontinuation of your supplemental estrogen may correct this situation. Discuss these issues with your physician.

TABLE 11. ESTROGEN TESTS: RESULTS AND INTERPRETATION

Estrogen Screening Blood Tests	*What do my results mean?	How do my lab results affect my weight?
Total Serum Estrogens **Premenopausal**	Normal: 70 to 900 pg/ml Abnormal: Above 900 pg/ml	Excess fat settles in different parts of your body at different stages of your life, and estrogen is mostly responsible for this rearrangement. If you're in your thirties or forties, for example, fat heads to your hips and thighs; taking birth control pills can make this worse. In your fifties and sixties, weight gain can gradually shift to your waistline. With an excess of estrogen in your system, your body accumulates fat more readily due to a slowdown in your metabolism. Excess estrogen can also drive up your appetite and cause problems with water retention—two other reasons for weight gain. Your doctor may individually decide to include other specialized hormone tests, based on your specific issues. As always, discuss all your symptoms with your doctor.
Postmenopausal	Normal: 130 pg/ml Abnormal: Above 130 pg/ml	
Adult Male	Normal: 130 pg/ml or less Abnormal: Above 130 pg/ml	

* *Values may vary depending upon laboratory used and your age and gender.*

YOUR BODY TYPE AND WEIGHT LOSS RESISTANCE

In addition to the testing I have just described, there is also a simple visual test you or your doctor can do if you truly believe you are weight loss resistant. You can look at yourself in the mirror, and right away, get an important clue as to why you're not losing weight. How? Where fat is concentrated on your body can be an important visual indicator of weight loss resistance. As much as I know you hate doing this, take a hard look at your body (preferably in the buff) in a full-length mirror. Don't skip this, please don't!

Do you tend to gain weight around your waist, with a shape that resembles an apple? Or is your weight collected mostly on your hips and thighs, with a shape that resembles a pear?

Making this simple observation and deciding whether your shape tends to be an apple body type or a pear body type is a practical yet amazing tool that has been used by physicians since the 1980s to interpret what's going on inside the human body. The location of the fat on your body tells you and your doctor whether you might be weight loss resistant, and what might be behind it.

For example, apple body types have trouble metabolizing carbohydrates. This may signal excess insulin production. In an attempt to clear sugar from the bloodstream, your body overproduces insulin. Fat cells in your abdominal area are particularly sensitive to insulin, and so you tend to gain fat around your midsection. In addition, when your metabolism slows down due to a sluggish thyroid, fat will accumulate at and above your waistline, as well as in other parts of your body.

When your body stores fat around your hips and thighs—the pear body type—this can be a visual indicator of estrogen imbalance, since a symptom of this imbalance is a pattern of lower-body fat distribution. Fat stored in the hips and thighs is more resistant to weight loss efforts.

An underactive thyroid is not associated with a specific body type. However, it will worsen weight gain around your hips and thighs if you have an estrogen imbalance. What's more, it will promote even greater fat accumulation around your waist if you also suffer from any metabolic imbalances. To add insult to injury, taking medications that have the side effect of weight gain can compound weight loss resistance in an underactive thyroid, Metabolic Syndrome, or estrogen imbalance.

OVERCOMING WEIGHT LOSS RESISTANCE

At this point, I hope you get it that there may be biochemical and physiological reasons for why you can't lose weight. It isn't a problem of eating too much. It isn't a matter of not exercising enough. It's not even a question of being emotionally weak. And it's not your fault.

If you know with certainty that you are in the category of weight loss resistance, though, this doesn't mean you're off the hook. This doesn't mean you can sit out the rest of the game. This doesn't mean you can ease up on your weight-management efforts, not use all seven keys, and have your cake and eat it, too. What it does mean is that you must begin to do different things in terms of your diet, your lifestyle, and the medical management of your condition, to prevent your weight and your health from getting totally out of control.

Finding out that you are weight loss resistant does not sentence you to a lifetime of obesity. It indicates only that your body has changed in some medically significant way. With the knowledge you have acquired through medical testing, you must now do something different in order to manage your weight. Although the treatment of weight loss resistance is beyond the scope of this book, I do not want to leave you in the lurch, without answers or solutions.

Because apple and pear body types have unique metabolic needs, one important step to take, in consultation with your physician, is to consider the use of specific nutritional supplements. Added to your daily routine, nutritional supplements will help you manage weight loss resistance not by directly fighting fat, but by helping to restore your body's metabolic balance.

There are supplements with scientifically researched levels of ingredients that can help you take better control of your weight, as long as you follow a nutritional plan like I have outlined and get regular exercise. Among the most important of these are specific vitamins, minerals, and herbs found in scientific research to have a significant impact on blood sugar control and metabolism. In Table 12 (page 262), you'll find information on these nutrients, including beneficial dosages, and which ones to use according to your body type. Each of these nutrients has solid clinical evidence (and a record of safety) behind it. Some of these you may recognize; others may be totally unfamiliar to you. As you and your physician decide which supplements to use, aim for products that supply these nutrients at the levels recommended in the table.

When you look over this list, you may be wondering, "Good grief, are you saying I have to take a fistful of pills every day?" No. The reason is that many of these nutrients, such as chromium, iodine, and vanadium, are already found in high-potency multivita-

TABLE 12. NUTRITIONAL SUPPLEMENTS FOR THE WEIGHT LOSS RESISTANT

Beneficial Roles of Selected Vitamins and Minerals In Weight Loss Resistance			
Nutrient	**What It Is**	***Beneficial Daily Dosages**	**Body Type**
Chromium	A mineral that helps maintain blood sugar levels within a normal range	200 mcg	Apple or Pear
Iodine	A mineral component of thyroid hormones	75 mcg	Apple or Pear
Magnesium	A mineral involved in more than 400 metabolic reactions in your body	400 mg	Apple or Pear
Selenium	A mineral that helps protect cells from damage	140 mcg	Apple or Pear
Vitamin C	A powerful antioxidant that protects cells against damage	500 mg	Apple or Pear
Vitamin E	A powerful antioxidant that guards cells and other tissues in the body	200 IU	Apple or Pear
Other Potentially Beneficial Nutrients			
Coenzyme Q10	A naturally occurring compound required for the production of energy in the body	100 mg	Apple or Pear
Conjugated Linoleic Acid (CLA)	A natural fatty acid found in safflower oil that may reduce the deposit of excess body fat and increase the ratio of lean body mass to fat, when combined with a low-calorie diet and exercise	2000 mg	Apple or Pear

Nutrient	What It Is	*Beneficial Daily Dosages	Body Type
Green tea extract	A metabolism-support herb	270 mg	Pear
L-Carnitine	A vitamin-like compound, made naturally by your body, involved in fat metabolism	100 mg	Apple or Pear
Omega-3 Fatty Acids	Healthy fats found naturally in fish, that support healthy body membranes and heart health	500 mg	Apple or Pear
Soy Isoflavones	Plant compounds that may promote heart health	50 mg	Pear
Vanadium	A mineral needed in small amounts by the body; helps maintain blood sugar levels within a normal range	10 mcg	Apple

* mcg-micrograms; mg-milligrams; IU-International Units

min–mineral supplements; others are available in combination in special metabolism-support supplements. So in reality you'd be taking far fewer pills than you might think.

Supplemental nutrients should never be used in place of a healthy lifestyle, behavioral control, or needed medical treatment. Miracle cures for weight loss they are not. But if you are genuinely weight loss resistant, there is sufficient scientific evidence to demonstrate that they may help you, along with diet and exercise.

Taking supplements is just one piece of your overall medical strategy, however. There is so much more you must do in terms of medical and lifestyle management. In Table 13 (page 264), you will find a synopsis of important medical and lifestyle strategies that are required to manage weight loss resistance and get you losing weight again.

When you work with this knowledge, harvesting the information and facts on these pages, your attempts at managing your weight are no longer a discouraging proposition because you have gotten no-kidding-real about what is actually happening in your body. Yes, you've got significant medical problems to correct. Yes, you've got challenges. And hopefully, you're willing to make choices to change them.

TABLE 13. MEDICAL AND LIFESTYLE STRATEGIES FOR THE WEIGHT LOSS RESISTANT

BODY TYPE	CONDITION	STRATEGIES
Apple or Pear	*Underactive thyroid*	Take thyroid medication as prescribed by your physician. This is the most important treatment strategy. Support medical treatment with an optimally healthful eating plan such as the High-Response Cost, High Yield Food Plan and nutritional supplements. Adopt an exercise program that includes weight training to keep your metabolism running in high gear; or a low-impact exercise program of tai chi or yoga if your physical energy is not yet up to par. Keep life stress under control so as not to aggravate thyroid problems.
Apple	*Metabolic Syndrome*	Fine-tune your diet to be low in fat and sugar and high in natural foods that supply plenty of vitamins and minerals, as the High-Response Cost, High Yield Food Plan suggests. Talk to your physician about whether taking supplemental vitamins and minerals will help improve your metabolic profile. Begin a regular exercise program that incorporates both aerobics and weight training in order to effectively burn pounds from your abdominal region. Eliminate addictive behavior such as smoking and alcohol abuse from your life; both aggravate Metabolic Syndrome and its associated symptoms. Reduce the stress in your life to a manageable level. Stress activates hormonal imbalances that lead to weight gain around the waist. Take medications if your physician prescribes them.

BODY TYPE	CONDITION	STRATEGIES
Pear	*Estrogen imbalance*	Increase the amount of fiber in your diet.
		Incorporate more soy foods into your diet most days to help naturally balance your body's hormone levels. Add to your diet a regimen of supplemental nutrients for metabolic support. A basic vitamin–mineral formula as a daily supplement can go a long way toward correcting possible deficiencies caused by supplemental hormones.
		Engage in a program of regular exercise to reduce body fat (which manufactures estrogen).
		Discuss with your physician what medical alternatives exist for hormonal replacement therapy (HRT).

When so much is at stake—your weight, your health, your self-esteem—you've got to do something about it. As I often say, life rewards action. You cannot passively place your health in the hands of your doctor and expect to be fixed like a car that needs a tune-up. You have to take the initiative and follow through in order to get your weight back in line. I know that is a tall order, but I'm letting you know without equivocation: that is exactly what you must do because your weight, your health, and your very life depend on it.

Once you begin to take action, you will gain a whole new control over the way you look, the way you feel, and the way you perform. The years of frustration and guilt over not reaching your goals will finally be over, and you will be able to attain a stable, comfortable, and close-to-perfect weight. It will take some effort and commitment on your part, but once you get going, the whole experience will be like taking the blindfold off and living your life as it should be.

I want to get you excited about getting your weight back in control, so that you can live differently. There is a remarkable power you can wield against weight loss resistance, if you are willing to work with your physician and comply with the proper treatment. Once you do: expect your pounds to swiftly vanish. Expect to feel healthier than you have in years. Expect to improve the quality of your life, and possibly even save it.

12

Weight Is Managed, Not Cured

It's not about what you tried to do, it's about the results. Life is a full contact sport, and there's a score up on the board.
—DR. PHIL

With the seven keys to permanent weight loss, you are now well equipped to keep shedding pounds until you arrive at a healthy, desirable size and the process of losing your excess weight winds down to its natural end. You have now within you every tool, all the know-how, the focus, the clarity, and the motivation necessary to succeed.

But let me be brutally honest with you: the vast majority of people who eventually reach their target weight do not retain that goal. Did you know, in fact, that there are just as many people trying to lose weight as there are people who are considered obese? The rate of obesity and the number of "dieters" in America are climbing in parallel!

Obviously, a lot of people just aren't staying at their goal weight. And the major reason, in my opinion, has to do with something called *instinctual drift*. A story I often use when teaching people about instinctual drift is the fable of the scorpion and the turtle. Being unable to swim, a scorpion pleaded with a turtle to carry him across a river. "No way!" bellowed the turtle. "You'll sting me in the neck while I'm swimming, and I'll drown."

The scorpion countered, "If I were to sting you, we'd both drown. So why would I sting you?"

"You're right," said the turtle. "Hop on." The scorpion climbed on the turtle's back and across the river they went. About halfway over, the scorpion stung the turtle in the neck. As they both sank to the bottom, the turtle moaned, "Why did you do that?"

To which the scorpion answered, "I couldn't help it. It's just my nature."

You see: instinctual drift is the tendency for all organisms, under certain conditions, to revert to their natural tendencies. You take a wild animal that has survived for centuries as a predator, artificially modify its behavior by trying to tame it, and then you are shocked when it reverts to its genetic programming and eats its master for lunch. This animal isn't being savage; it's just doing what is natural for it to do. We humans may be smarter (or not), but we operate in much the same way.

It's like this: you have a long history of learned and overlearned behaviors—in the way you eat, the way you think, the way you feel, and the way you act—so overlearned, in fact, that they have become second-nature habits to which you instinctually drift when under stress or pressure. Whenever you're not actively managing your weight, your health, and your life with a great degree of awareness and programming. Second-nature habits do not change quickly. That's why there is so much truth in the familiar saying, "Old habits die hard."

Your past behavior, with these deeply ingrained patterns of thinking, feeling, and acting, is unfortunately the best predictor of your future behavior. For most people, this means that if you have tried to lose weight before but failed, you will most likely fail in the future. If you have been an overeater every day for years and years, then the best prediction is that you will continue to be an overeater this year. If you have been habitually inactive every day for most of your adult life, then the best prediction is that you will be inactive again this year. That's your big burden; that's your great obstacle right now in your journey toward permanent weight loss and control. The flow of life in general, and your lifestyle in particular, will conspire to suck you back into the unproductive, unhealthy way of living that you are working so hard to escape.

But stop right here: this does not have to be true for you. Now that you know something about why you eat and why you are overweight, and what you can do about it, you have the wherewithal to get on the right track and head in a different direction. If your history of overeating predicts your future and you want a new future—one with a healthy weight and a stronger self-image—then you begin by creating a new history. Every day that you use the seven keys to permanent weight loss, this has the important effect of building a new and positive history for you. Days turn into weeks, weeks into months, months into years, and your relevant past behavior is healthy and productive—and thus the most accurate prediction for the future becomes more of the same.

Understand, too, that success is a moving target, and that in an ever-changing world, if after reading this book you implement all of the keys and steps that you learned and came to accept, your weight will very likely be just where you want it or moving closer. Of course, I will be happy for you. But you should not believe that you will have fixed your weight problem 100 percent. When you decide to take charge of your weight, there is still a lot of work ahead. It takes effort, action, and commitment to shake free of your past negative programming. There is still a part of you that is comfortable in these old ways of being and doing, and it is that part of you that maybe doesn't want things to change and will put up a good fight.

You have spent much of your life working real hard at staying real fat and creating a lifestyle that supports being heavy. You have set up that lifestyle, based upon those self-defeating parts of yourself that cause you to lose control over your weight—and believe me, the simple fact that you now recognize how you have been sabotaging yourself does not fix the problem. You must go through many years of maintaining your weight loss to get over so many years of staying so heavy. What your weight is five years from now will be a function of how well you actively manage these things from now until then.

I hope I'm not knocking a dent in your enthusiasm. Believe me, because of the keys you have learned in this book, you are now part of a group of people who know what it takes to get results that last. But there's a big difference between knowing and doing, between being capable of lasting change and living a commitment to change. What you're about to face is no different from someone who walks into a dark movie theater. At first it's so dark that you can't see where you are going. But as you find a seat and settle into it, the darkness seems to clear and you can see again. In fact, you can see almost normally. But never forget that you are in darkness. That is the same predicament in which you find yourself if you lose your commitment to weight management and stop taking action. You'll be plunged back in a dim, dark world, where poor choices and self-defeating behavior become the norm again. All of your past history, all of your old habits, all of everything you threw off, continue to darken your world. If you remain there, you will begin to think that this is normal for you and start conforming to your old way of living. It is not normal. I want you to be part of the group who have the courage and determination to stay in the light.

I hope it has been exciting for you to operate under the specific programming that I have given you, completing your audits and questionnaires and using the keys and steps to permanent weight loss. But this process is not yet over. There are danger zones behind every one of these doors, where you and your ability to control your weight are extremely vulnerable.

For me to state this any less emphatically would be to cheat you. That's why, as we come to the end of this book, I want to make sure that you are aware of these danger zones so that you know how to handle them, and hang on to what you have worked so hard to achieve. What follows is a hard look at the most common danger zones that will bubble up in your life as you move forward from here. Have the commitment to get real about these danger zones, and you can take control.

THE DANGER ZONE OF DISAPPOINTMENT

Okay, maybe you're fantasizing that once you reach your target weight, the new you will have a new job, a new girlfriend or boyfriend, and a new life altogether. Then you wake up one morning, thin, trim, and fit, and none of these dreams materializes. They don't come true because that is not the world you live in day to day. Not everyone loves you now that you are thin. You didn't get a raise. Your marriage is still on the rocks. You were miserable fat; now you're miserable skinny.

The moment this disappointment hits you, there's an automatic tendency to think, "What the heck . . . was it really worth the trouble to lose all that weight and still have the same old life?" There's a harsh truth to take into account here: your disenchantment gives you a face-saving excuse to keep failing at life, and so what happens is that you revert to your old thoughts, your old feelings, your old behaviors—and, eventually, your old fat self. When you expect life's problems to vanish when you achieve your target goal, you are not being realistic, and you increase your odds of quitting the whole deal.

Or maybe you look around at other skinny people—your coworker who has a great body, your neighbor who looks terrific in a bikini, or your brother with his rippling biceps—and you imagine that their lives must be so perfect, because after all, if they're in great shape, their lives must be in great shape. Now, the truth of the matter is, elevating such people to some pedestal of perfection is a total crock; there is no perfect life. It doesn't exist.

I've been humbled in my life with the opportunity to interview many famous people, and I have often asked them, "How does it feel to be so famous?" You may be surprised to learn that, invariably, the famous compare themselves to other famous people—stars as glamorous as they are—and tell me, "I don't feel the way they look."

To them, "famous" doesn't feel like it looks. It doesn't feel glamorous, it doesn't feel successful, it doesn't feel special. "Famous" never feels from the inside out what it looks like from the outside in. Neither does "thin."

If you expect to feel like other people look, setting up such unrealistic expectations for what life will be like as a thin person, then you are living in a dream world. In doing so, you guarantee failure because the expectations you seem to be holding are so terribly unrealistic. Thus, it is important as you use the keys to lose weight, and then to maintain that weight loss, that you be realistic about what you expect of yourself and your life.

If you are to avoid this danger zone and not retreat to old patterns of living that kept you fat, but maintain your weight loss for a lifetime, there is no room in your life for fantasy or fiction. You can help yourself if your expectations about what will happen when you achieve your target weight are realistic rather than naïve. Yes, you must hold yourself to high standards, but these standards must be realistic. Do not kid yourself about the scope or demands of your weight challenges, nor of your life as a healthier, more fit person. Know who you are and what you can realistically achieve and build from that truth.

The Danger Zone of Fixed Fat Beliefs

If you have been heavy for very long, you may have a perception of yourself as a fat person, even though you have dropped several sizes and plenty of pounds. That perception is composed of something called *fixed beliefs*, a negative self-perception that you have decided is true and accurate about you. Some of your fixed beliefs may be rooted as far back as childhood, others may have developed more recently. Whatever their origin, many of these fixed beliefs are products of the fat image you hold of yourself—hardened assumptions you've formed about yourself over your history of being overweight, however wrong or outdated now. Because you are or were overweight, you believe you can't do certain things, you don't deserve something, or you are not qualified. You believe these things are true, and so you accept them and live with them. To illustrate what I'm talking about, here are some typical fixed beliefs that people with weight problems have shared with me:

I'm just not worthy.

I can't reach my weight loss goals.

I will never come out on top at work because I'm fat.

That's for thin people.

I feel too conspicuous to go out.

I won't get the job.

I don't deserve anything better than what I've got.

I can't make myself look any nicer.

Most beliefs like these are limiting beliefs. You can think of them like internal straitjackets, imposing such restrictions on you that the possibility of ever viewing yourself as anything but fat or flawed seems somehow out of reach. Whether your limiting beliefs are like those just listed, or something very different, in this psychological state you will overlook important changes in yourself (like weight loss) that would negate the beliefs. You are cheating yourself if such beliefs have their hooks in you. As one who has counseled thousands of overweight patients, I have seen far too many people locked in that familiar but frustrating pattern of weight loss followed by weight gain, because they still think of themselves as overweight. As dwellers in this zone, they remain at very high risk of regaining the fat they never psychologically shed. Even if they do lose weight, they have trouble telling themselves that they deserve more and that they want more, because they are being held back so dramatically by their limiting beliefs. People will limit themselves so dramatically, it's just amazing.

Recognize, too, that you may be getting certain payoffs from some of your limiting beliefs. As you lose weight and become thin, a large part of your physical appearance is leaving, and this can be threatening and scary. Although for years you have wanted desperately to shed this weight and keep it off, when it begins to disappear, you may feel uncomfortable in your new, smaller body. Staying fat has been working for you in some fashion. Since it is a law of life that people do what works, your obesity has been affording you some type of payoff. Maybe you have used your obesity as insulation against attention from the opposite sex, neutralizing your sexual attractiveness. Maybe you have used your weight as an occupational buffer zone, to hide your femininity and protect yourself from the attention of male peers at work. Maybe you have used your obesity as an excuse for your failures. You have told yourself you didn't get the job, date the guy or gal, or sign up for the class because you were just too overweight.

As your shape changes, you may miss your insulation, your buffer zone, and your excuses, and understandably feel ill at ease and ready to push the panic button. It is this discomfort that makes you compromise; it is this discomfort that causes you to work at cross-purposes with your healthy goals. If you try to manage your weight from behind these defenses, you will fail. So now is definitely not the time to panic or disconnect.

Understand too that if you have been overweight for many years, it will take time to change your "fat mind-set" and your "fixed fat beliefs" about yourself. You must learn to become comfortable in your new, trimmer body, and at the same time you must learn to dump your "psychological fat." You can't do this unless you start acting like the thin, fit person you really are. By acting like the way you look, you give yourself the chance to experience the positive feelings that follow from that behavior. Even if it doesn't feel completely right, you can move in that direction with some simple but positive actions. Before you know it, new, confident, and truthful beliefs about yourself will become the rule rather than the exception. Some of the ways to help shed your psychological fat and get comfortable in your own skin include: looking at your reflection in the mirror more often to acclimate yourself to your new shape and image; facing with courage those situations you formerly feared (wearing a bathing suit, trying on new clothes, or going to parties and other social outings); staying with your exercise program in order to appreciate your own strength and feel good about your body; and tuning in to negative self-talk about your body and replacing it with accurate and affirming thoughts.

Be patient with yourself as you go through this process, because it takes time. Think about changing your limiting beliefs as remodeling a house that doesn't fit your lifestyle anymore. In order to live comfortably in your home again, sometimes you have to strip away old wallpaper, tear down obstructive walls, replace outdated fixtures, or repair structural cracks. So it is with beliefs: you have to peel away whatever fixed assumptions you have, dispose of their payoffs, demolish old limiting beliefs inside you that are telling you that you're worthless and not deserving of success, discard them, and replace them with new knowledge and genuine insight. Only then can you move on to new ways of thinking about yourself that will yield new payoffs. Only then can you live peacefully and comfortably in your new, transformed body.

If you really want to change your limiting beliefs, don't do it halfway. That dog won't hunt. Not even close. Whatever the messages in your head, the beliefs and payoffs they provide lead to unsuccessful behavior, which threatens your weight and your ability to control it. If you fail to address them, you will compromise your ability to adapt what you're learning in this book to achieve permanent weight loss and control.

THE DANGER ZONE OF RELAXED EFFORT

I realize that there is a natural tendency to relax immediately after reading a book such as this, or keeping its techniques in play. You have made real progress, but now is not the time to relax. This is the time to make sure you continue to use the seven keys over the long term, in order to counteract the strong negative pull of your environment and the real-world challenges you will face in trying to manage your weight.

Having lost a lot of weight and even reached your goal weight, you may feel that you can handle things now and that you can let down your guard. But as the title of this chapter states: *Weight is managed, not cured*. You must never relax your watchfulness over your thoughts, feelings, and actions. Your guiding objective must always be to manage your weight, and indeed, your overall health, with a keen sense of alertness.

Managing your weight from this point forward involves making a commitment to something psychologists call "self-monitoring," a process of keeping tabs on your progress and performance, in order to prevent self-defeating behaviors from regaining even a toehold in your life. Not surprisingly, evidence demonstrates that people who regularly self-monitor their behavior are more successful at maintaining their weight losses than those who are inconsistent.

Failure to self-monitor, in my opinion, is one of the top reasons why people allow their weight to creep back on. They don't recognize even the smallest weight gain or snugness in their clothes because they don't want it to be true, and as a result, they choose to deny warning signs that otherwise would cause them to take immediate corrective action. By refusing to acknowledge that you are again out of control, not eating right, not exercising enough, and not managing your behavior as you should, you let valuable time slip away, and with it precious opportunities to take important and timely coping steps. You must acknowledge the presence of warning signs so that you can make a conscious effort to offset or control that condition. What you do not acknowledge is only going to get worse until you do.

In order to avoid this danger zone, make a deal with yourself right now: you will weigh yourself with reasonable frequency—at least once a week—though not obsessively, to stay on target. Do this at the same time each week because your weight fluctuates throughout the day, and you can weigh more at night than you do in the morning. Give yourself an acceptable weight-gain range, say 5 pounds or so, that you will not let yourself exceed. Promise yourself you will not self-destruct if the scale moves up a few pounds, but instead make this a priority for action-oriented repair. Check your weight and shape against the Body Weight Standards and the Body Shape Standards in Chapter 2. At the same time, keep a food journal and record your exercise progress in your workout diary.

As you prepare to go forward, let me encourage you to look back at the considerable work you've already done. It's perfectly acceptable, and in fact, a good idea to "re-audit" your internal dialogue, emotional eating, stress, environment, nutrition habits, exercise, and support level. Maybe it helps to reexamine yourself in these areas and retake these tests in two, four, six months, a year or more from now. I believe that after doing some re-auditing, it would be fair to say you are a different person from the one who started this book. Your weight and your health have started moving in the right direction, and for sure, your self-knowledge has advanced much farther down the road. But if you don't require much of yourself in this area of self-monitoring, your ability to maintain your goal weight will be weakened considerably. I'm not trying to drag you down; I just want you to get real.

THE DANGER ZONE OF CRISIS

Because living is hardly painfree, never will your life be without crisis. It is not a matter of if; it is a matter of when. When a crisis hits—whether it is a bankruptcy, a divorce, a serious illness or accident, or a death—you need to be doubly careful because the desire to escape the painful realities of that crisis may override your commitment to managing your weight. When in a crisis mode, you push all your priorities off the list and you suspend all the rules, because, you tell yourself, it is okay to get some right-now relief from your pain. Once this type of emotionally charged thinking enters the mix, your self-management skills simply fall apart. When that happens, you have shifted your momentum back into reverse, and you will keep your destructive behaviors revived and recurring. When food and unhealthy behaviors become your escape hatch, you sometimes end up doing nothing to resolve the crisis, because you have incapacitated yourself. Quite possibly you will make the situation worse. But let's get real here: isn't a crisis a time when you need to really concentrate on healthy behavior for energy, for focus, and for clarity of thinking? Isn't it? Really managing yourself during a crisis means that you will not live reactively, you will not let your life slide, and you will not let the crisis paralyze your life.

Your best chance to take back control is to have a consciously designed plan in place for dealing with the crises that will inevitably erupt in your life. If you have a plan and the courage, commitment, and energy to execute it, you will overcome the tough stuff. The plan I'm talking about involves perfecting the coping skills you have adopted and put into practice while learning about the seven keys to permanent weight loss. In other words, stay with whatever has improved your life thus far, and move yourself up the performance ladder in order to stimulate even stronger coping responses for what lies ahead. If, for example, you have learned the fundamentals of yoga as a tension-reducing activity, take it to another level by studying advanced forms of yoga. Be willing to get out of your comfort zones and require more of yourself physically, mentally, emotionally, and behaviorally. Never tell yourself beforehand that something is impossible, nor set limits on your efforts. Be willing to leave behind the safe, unchallenging, and familiar ways of doing things in order to have more. Step up and do this, and enjoy the rewards of physical and psychological fitness that flow from your willingness to stretch and reach. When you do, you will find a new level of personal power. You will have matured to a new level of functioning that will give you the courage to make choices that make you feel good about yourself, no matter what arises in your life.

When a crisis hits—and trust me, it will—I want you to be able to say:

This is exactly what Dr. Phil said would happen, and I will not be ambushed by this situation. In the past, a crisis was a cue for dis-

integration, now it's a cue for coping. I am prepared because I have positive ways to cope with crisis, rather than react by choosing foods and behavior that put my physical and emotional health at risk. I will handle this in a rational, manageable fashion, and not make foolish choices. I am in control, and I have no desire to jeopardize that control.

Footnote: I strongly believe that while crises can be trying and they can be terrible, they can ultimately strengthen us. There is a fitting analogy in the giant sequoia, the tallest of all living trees. Paradoxically, this majestic tree grows best when small wildfires periodically clear the forest, providing sunlight and soil nutrients to nourish the trees. Yes, the fires may wound the trees deeply, but ultimately they ensure their survival. Likewise, a crisis is not to our detriment, but to our development.

THE DANGER ZONE OF REWARD AND PUNISHMENT

As you use the seven keys to permanent weight loss and act on their steps, be alert to the possibility that you may want to "reward" yourself in ways that totally negate every positive move you've made up to this point. When halfhearted about changing their lives, people tend to default to their undesirable behaviors, and use these behaviors as a reward system in various situations. If you do this, you have wrongly defined and mislabeled the concept of "reward."

A good example of this is the guy who leaves work every night, and heads to Happy Hour, where he has several martinis to reward himself for a hard day's work, instead of going home to spend meaningful time with his family. Going to Happy Hour feels rewarding for the brief time he is there, but it has a hugely negative impact right away as the alcohol kills off millions of brain cells, or the next day, when he is too hung-over to work productively or maybe even show up for work. It will have a hugely negative impact a few months or a few years from now, when his family life, his health, his career, and, indeed, his overall standard of living are sacrificed. It seems stranger than fiction: how could anyone think that the sick behavior described here qualifies as a reward? It's anything but. It's punishment.

Just as with the guy in the above scenario, you may feel like doing something dumb, too—for instance, "rewarding" yourself with a banana split after complying with this plan. Don't do that. Please don't do that. It is certainly not a reward, when you have worked for months to reconstitute your mind, body, and spirit. Don't choose to make spontaneous, hedonistic choices that can wreck your weight and your health. Consider what is lost by that illogical, nonreaching, destructive behavior: all it does is erase days, weeks, and months of productive, healthy work, and you're back to square one.

If you wish to reward yourself for positive behavior, do so appropriately, with choices and actions that are nonfood-related. When you start changing the rewards, you start changing the consequences. I recall a patient of mine who established a positive reward system and found a higher degree of self-worth in the process. She told me, "In the past, I used to reward myself for finishing a big project by going out for dinner and drinks. But that was the wrong approach for me, one that was ultimately depriving me of health, self-respect, and an attractive appearance. I decided to reward myself in other ways— by having facials, manicures, or massages. I feel like I'm taking better care of myself as a result, and it has done wonders for my self-image and self-confidence."

When you redefine reward and punishment in your life, as this woman did, you lift your self-management skills to a higher plane. When you take care of yourself in healthy, healing ways, your weight will become so much easier to manage and maintain, and you will have the energy and motivation to do even more of what needs to be done.

THE DANGER ZONE OF ISOLATION

Next to exercise, having the support you need has often been cited as one of the most important factors in managing and maintaining weight loss. Yes, I know I'm beating the drums on this, but you need a supportive network of people in your life. And you need them more than ever after you reach your target weight. Don't isolate yourself, thinking, "Now that I'm thin, I don't need an accountability source, and I don't need a coach, a teammate, a cheerleader, or an umpire."

Wrong! If you hope to keep your weight off, you have to live the motto that "a healthy lifestyle loves company," and surround yourself with friends, family, and other social resources who subscribe to the same motto—people who lift you up, rather than hold you down. Put another way, never dissolve the supporting team you put together in the seventh key. Let me tell you why this is so important: it's just a psychological truth that behavioral change is more successful if it is supported by a caring, loyal, and encouraging network of like-minded people who want you to win. As you face the future, not only should you choose what you eat, how you act, and what you think and feel, you must also choose your support circle. If you truly want to change, surround yourself with people who want you to succeed, and you will succeed.

Avoiding these danger zones is of great importance to managing your weight. While you may have some strikeouts, you must not let them discourage or deter you. If it takes one swing of the bat, fine. If it takes ten, that's okay, too. Learn from these things, and live what you have learned. You have started to transform your life, and there is a noticeable difference in how you engage the world. You have changed your momentum to create a life of energy, meaning, and purpose. There are really no limits to what you can now achieve, nothing can push you down, because you look better, feel better, and live better. Continue to press on with an optimistic spirit.

From Dr. Phil to You

Weight Control
That Lasts

In many ways, the end of this book is just the beginning: the beginning of a brand new way of living for you. When you do things differently, giving up those parts of your life that have been self-defeating for those which are self-affirming, your weight, your health, and your life change dramatically. You acquire self-discipline and strength. You gain a new perspective. You enjoy the positive results of accepting and liking yourself once more. And you find new meaning to your life and hope for your future.

You have wanted to lose weight for a very long time, and you must admit that never before have you had a better shot at doing it until now. I haven't given you a magic diet. I haven't told you that you can get skinny in seven days. I haven't promised you a metabolic miracle.

What I have told you is the real deal: that to change your weight, to achieve permanent weight loss, you have to be totally, consciously in charge of yourself and everything you do, think, and feel. And you have to use that control to create the healthy "you" that you deserve to be and have. If you have worked through this book sincerely, you are now ready to live this new life and experience the joy that will gush forth from it.

With the seven keys to permanent weight loss, you now have a concrete plan of action in place for living a healthier, richer, and fuller life. The more you put into this plan, as you go forward the more you will get out of it. When it comes to managing your weight for a lifetime, make use of everything you've been given here. Remember all the steps and tools we've talked about throughout this book. If you ever find yourself slipping backwards, take command of the situation by using the seven keys. Reaching your get-real weight, when you have the keys, follow the steps, and avoid all the danger zones, should be a one-way trip, and you will never, ever, have to carry with you the baggage of unwanted fat.

I believe that what works in your life works because you make it work. You succeed because you make the right choices, you choose the right attitude, and you enact the right behavior to generate the right results. It is you who must create the life you want. And the choice is yours to make.

What matters now is that you continue to build this life for yourself, a life that with each passing day will bring you health, energy, confidence, peace of mind that cannot be disturbed, and a spirit that soars. If you can do this—and you can—then you will have what you want because you made the choices, you accomplished what was required, and you reached for the best that was within you.

Here's to you.

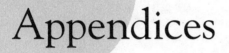

Appendices

Appendix A

Stress Relief and Relaxation Script

Find the quietest, most comfortable, and most private place you can. Ideally, you want to set aside a solid thirty minutes, during which no one can bother you. This may be very difficult for some of you because of the demands of the telephone, your kids, commitments, and a thousand other things you may have to do. Usually, it is when you finally find an opportunity to relax that your memory begins to intrude, reminding you of everything else you "should be" doing. Psychologically, this is only your ego attempting to wrest command of your attention, or another part of your mind attempting to prevent you from relaxing.

Disregard these messages so that you can take control and pursue your relaxation. Amazingly, thirty minutes of true relaxation equates to two full hours of sleep for restoration. Thus, this all-important thirty minutes should be safeguarded from outside demands.

As you begin to take steps to relax, expect distractions and emotive responses to emerge from the inner recesses of your brain. To minimize these internal reactions, I highly recommend that you find some soothing music to accompany your relaxation, or read the instructions over a tape player so that you can be "guided" instead of having to remember the steps. It might also be useful for you to include some of your own imagery—a vacation spot or a tranquil setting—whatever internal scenes help you relax best. Include these thoughts in your relaxation sequence.

To begin, start by focusing on your breathing: not to change it but just to become aware of how it feels to breathe in and to breathe out. Feel the experience from inside your body. As you take some time to look inside and feel your breaths, let me explain that your out-breath allows your body to release anything it no longer needs or wants, such as dead air, tension, carbon dioxide, poisons, and even some kinds of virus and bacteria. So focus on letting go of everything you want to let go, especially stress, fear, and any other destabilizing emotions. Just let them go with your next out-breath. For a few moments, practice letting go of any tension, stress, feelings, or thoughts that you just don't need right now. Let them go.

Next, I want you to know that when you let these things go with your out-breath, you are replacing that space with good, nurturing air with your in-breath. Visualize that good air coming into your body and healing whatever needs physical restoration. Send that air to anywhere in your body and feel the love and caring you are giving yourself right now. Bring it into yourself. Practice this for a little while.

What you need to do next is to balance these in-breaths with the out-breaths, so that you will feel soothing relaxation and balance coming into your body. Practice breathing in to a count of seven, 1-2-3-4-5-6-7, now breathe out, 1-2-3-4-5-6-7, in-breath, 1-2-3-4-5-6-7, and out-breath 1-2-3-4-5-6-7. Count for yourself for each in-breath and out-breath for at least five minutes.

Note to yourself that you are balancing your out-breaths and in-breaths, letting the bad stress and tension leave your body, and allowing the good nurturing air to come in. You are releasing the negative poisons and bringing the healing forces in.

From here, you need to bring the rest of your body into sync with this response. Can you feel your heart beat? Can you feel your pulse, or the heartbeat in your stomach or somewhere else? Use the number of heartbeats to balance your breathing. Take a moment to see what works best for you. It may not be seven beats between the breaths. It may be four or three or five. Whatever feels right, begin to breathe out and in to the same number of heartbeats. Give yourself a moment to regulate that balance for yourself. Do this for five minutes by yourself.

Before you stop, do a quick review of your body, following this sequence:

Are your feet more relaxed? If not, relax them with your breathing.

Are your legs more relaxed? If not, relax them with your breathing.

Is your pelvis more relaxed? If not, relax it with your breathing.

Is your stomach more relaxed? If not, relax it with your breathing.

Is your chest more relaxed? If not, relax it with your breathing.

Is your back more relaxed? If not, relax it with your breathing.

Are your arms more relaxed? If not, relax them with your breathing.

Are your hands more relaxed? If not, relax them with your breathing.

Is your mind more relaxed? If not, relax it with your breathing.

Do this, all in sync with your breathing.

Continue to go through the rest of your day, and if you need to relax or take your mind off food, stop and start this same breathing–relaxation sequence.

Food Lists

What follows is a partial list of foods to guide you in your decision making, food selection, and meal planning. In the first list, I've placed an asterisk next to the foods that are truly high-response cost—foods that require effort for ingestion and/or preparation. Remember: high-response cost, high-yield foods support good eating habits and provide excellent nutrition.

The second food lists gives you low-response cost, low-yield foods—easy to ingest, easily accessible, and weak in nutritional quality. Keep in mind that these foods should be avoided, or at best limited in your diet, since they can exact a harmful cost on your body by paving the way to obesity, heart disease, diabetes, and other lifestyle-related diseases.

FOODS TO CHOOSE:

HIGH-RESPONSE COST, HIGH-YIELD FOODS

Proteins (fish, meat, plant proteins, poultry, shellfish): 3 servings

Dairy: 2 servings

Carbohydrates:
2 to 3 servings of starches (breads, grains, cereals, and/or starchy
    vegetables)
2 fruits
4 servings of vegetables

Fats: 1 serving

See page 183 for more information on the number of servings per day.

High-response Cost, High-yield Proteins

Fish (all baked or broiled unless otherwise noted)
*Bass
*Bluefish
*Cod
*Flounder
*Grouper
*Haddock
*Halibut
*Ocean perch
*Pollock
*Salmon, also grilled
    Canned
    Smoked
Sardines, canned in water, or in mustard or other nonfat sauce
*Swordfish, also grilled
*Trout
*Tuna, also grilled
    Canned, in water

Shellfish
Clams
    Canned
    *Steamed
Crab
    *Boiled or steamed
    Canned
    Imitation (surimi)
*Lobster, boiled or steamed
*Oysters
    Cooked, with a nonfat sauce
    Raw
*Scallops, broiled or steamed
*Shrimp, boiled or steamed

Poultry (all baked or roasted unless otherwise noted)
Chicken
    *Breast, no skin
    Canned
    *Ground, lean
*Cornish game hen, no skin
*Turkey
    Breast, no skin; also barbecued or smoked
    Ground, lean
    Sausage, lean

Meats (all broiled or grilled unless otherwise noted)
*Beef, well-trimmed of fat
    Ground, extra lean or lean
    Round (all cuts)
    Sirloin
    Tenderloin
    Top loin
*Lamb, well-trimmed of fat
    Chop
    Ribs
    Shoulder
Lunch meats
    Bologna, light (turkey)
    Ham, reduced-fat
    Reduced-fat or nonfat sandwich meats
*Pork, well-trimmed of fat
    Chop
    Roast
*Veal, rib chop, well-trimmed of fat

Plant Proteins
*Beans (such as black, garbanzo, kidney, pinto, white; see also
    Vegetables, Starchy, page 297)
Peanut butter, reduced-fat (use very sparingly)
*Soy burgers or hot dogs
*Tempeh
*Textured vegetable protein
Tofu

*Eggs
Liquid egg substitute
Whites
Whole (not cooked in fat)

Low-Fat Dairy Foods
Cheese, reduced-fat or nonfat
    Brick
    Cheddar
    Feta
    Mozzarella
    Parmesan
    Processed, reduced-fat
    Ricotta, part skim milk
    Swiss
    Cottage cheese
        Low-fat 2%
        Low-fat 1%
        Nonfat
Ice milk, fat-free and sugar-free
Milk
    1% (low-fat)
    2% (low-fat)
    Buttermilk, reduced-fat or nonfat
    *Nonfat milk reconstituted with water from instant powder
    Skim milk
    Soy milk
Yogurt, plain (unsweetened)
    Low-fat
    Nonfat

HIGH-RESPONSE COST, HIGH-YIELD CARBOHYDRATES

Breads and Bread Products
Bagels
    Oat bran
    Whole-wheat
Breads
    Cracked wheat

High-fiber (Branola)
Mixed grain
Oatmeal
Pita, whole-wheat
Pumpernickel
Raisin, enriched
Rye, light or dark
Whole-wheat
Crackers
Low-fat and whole-wheat varieties
Melba toast
English muffin, whole-wheat
Muffins
Bran, small
Whole-wheat, small
Rolls, whole-wheat
Tortillas, corn

Cereals
Cold cereals
*All-Bran
*All-Bran Extra Fiber
*Bran Buds
Bran Checks
Corn bran
Corn Chex
Fortified Oat Flakes
40% Bran Flakes
Fruit & Fibre
Fruitful Bran
Granola, low-fat
Grape-Nuts
Mueslix
100% Bran
Product 19
Raisin Bran
Rice Chex
Rice, puffed

     Shredded Wheat
     Special K
     Total
     *Wheat bran, raw (use 1–2 tablespoons, sprinkled on other cereals)
     Wheat Chex
     *Wheat germ, raw or toasted (use 1–2 tablespoons, sprinkled on
         other cereals)
     Wheat, puffed
Cooked Cereals (Starches)
     *Corn grits (hominy); enriched, regular or quick
     Corn grits, instant
     *Cream of Wheat, regular or quick
     Cream of Wheat, instant
     *Farina
     *Malt-O-Meal
     *Oat bran
     *Oatmeal, regular or quick
     Oatmeal, instant

Grain Products
*Cooked grains
     Aramanth
     Barley, pearl
     Bulgur wheat
     Couscous
     Millet
     Quinoa
*Pasta (with low-fat or nonfat sauce)
     Spinach
     Whole-wheat
*Rice
     Brown rice
     Wild rice

Vegetables, non-starchy (raw and/or cooked)
*Alfalfa sprouts
*Artichokes
     Fresh, boiled or steamed
     Frozen hearts or quarters
*Arugula

Asparagus
    Canned
        *Fresh
        *Frozen
*Bamboo shoots
Beans
    *String beans, fresh or frozen
    String beans, canned
    *Yellow snap beans, fresh or frozen
    Yellow snap beans, canned
Bean sprouts
    Canned
    *Fresh
Beets
    Canned
    *Fresh
*Beet greens, cooked
*Broccoli
    Cooked from fresh or frozen
    Raw
*Broccoflower
*Brussels sprouts, cooked from fresh or frozen
*Cabbage, fresh green or red
    Cooked
    Raw
Carrots
    Canned
    *Cooked from fresh or frozen
    Juice, canned or fresh
    *Raw
*Cauliflower
    Cooked from fresh or frozen
    Raw
*Celery, raw
*Collards, cooked from fresh or frozen
*Cucumbers, raw
*Eggplant (not fried)
*Endive
*Escarole

*Kale, cooked from fresh or frozen
*Leeks, cooked
*Lettuce, all varieties
Mushrooms
    Canned, drained
    *Cooked from fresh
    *Fresh, raw
*Mustard greens, cooked from fresh or frozen
*Okra, cooked from fresh or frozen
*Onions, cooked or raw
    Globe onions
    Pearl onions
    Shallots
    Spring—green—scallions
*Parsley
*Parsnips, cooked
Peas, green
    Canned
    *Cooked from fresh or frozen
Peas and carrots
    Canned
    *Cooked from fresh or frozen
Peppers, hot, all varieties
    Canned
    *Raw
*Peppers, sweet, green, red, and yellow
    Cooked
    Raw
*Rutabaga, cooked from fresh or frozen
Sauerkraut
Spinach
    Canned, drained
    *Cooked from fresh or frozen
    *Raw
*Squash, summer, cooked
*Succotash, fresh or frozen
Tomatoes
    Canned

*Cooked, fresh
*Raw, chopped or whole
Tomato products, canned
    Juice
    Paste
    Purée
    Sauce
*Turnips, cooked from fresh or frozen
*Turnip greens, cooked from fresh or frozen
Vegetable juice cocktail, canned
Vegetables, mixed
    Canned
    *Cooked frozen
*Water chestnuts
*Watercress
*Zucchini
    Cooked fresh
    Raw

Vegetables, starchy, cooked
Beans and legumes
    Black beans
        Canned
        *Cooked from dry
    Black-eyed peas
        Canned
        *Cooked from dry or frozen
    Chickpeas, canned
    Great Northern beans
        Canned
        *Cooked from dry
    Kidney beans
        Canned
        *Cooked from dry
    Lima beans
        Canned
        *Cooked from dry or frozen
    *Lentils, cooked from dry

*Navy beans, cooked from dry
Pinto beans
    Canned
      *Cooked from dry
*Soy beans, cooked from dry
*Split peas, green or yellow, cooked from dry
*Corn
    Canned (not creamed)
    Kernels, frozen
    On the cob, fresh or frozen
*Potato
    Baked, skin on (medium)
    Boiled, peeled
Pumpkin, canned
*Squash, winter, cooked from fresh or frozen
*Sweet potato, baked, skin on (medium)

Fruits
Apples
    *Dried
    *Fresh
    Sauce, unsweetened
Apricots
    Canned, juice or water pack
    *Dried
    *Fresh
Bananas
Blackberries
    *Fresh
    Frozen, unsweetened
Blueberries
    *Fresh
    Frozen, unsweetened
Cherries
    Canned, water pack
    *Dried
    *Fresh
*Cranberries, dried

*Figs, dried
Fruit cocktail, juice or water pack
Grapefruit
    Canned sections, juice pack
    *Fresh
*Grapes, fresh
*Kiwi fruit, fresh
*Lemons
*Limes
*Mangoes
*Melon
    Cantaloupe
    Casaba
    Honeydew
    Watermelon
*Nectarines, fresh
Oranges
    Canned sections, juice pack
    *Fresh
*Papayas, fresh
Peaches
    Canned, juice or water pack
    *Dried
    *Fresh
    Frozen, unsweetened
Pears
    Canned, juice or water pack
    *Dried
    *Fresh
Pineapple
    Canned, juice pack, chunks, crushed, slices, tidbits
    *Fresh, slices or chunks
Plums
    Canned, juice pack
    *Fresh
Prunes
    *Dried
    Stewed, unsweetened

*Raisins (limit to 1 packet or 2 tablespoons)
Raspberries
    *Fresh
    Frozen, unsweetened
Strawberries
    *Fresh
    Frozen, unsweetened
*Tangelos, fresh
*Tangerines, fresh

Fruit Juices
Acerola
Apple, unsweetened
Cranberry juice cocktail, low-calorie
Grape, unsweetened
Grapefruit, unsweetened
Orange, unsweetened
Pineapple, unsweetened
Prune, unsweetened

HIGH-RESPONSE COST, HIGH-YIELD FATS
(USE VERY SPARINGLY)

Fats and Oils
Canola oil
Flaxseed oil
Margarine, trans-free
Olive oil
Peanut oil
Safflower oil
Sesame oil
Sunflower oil
Vegetable oils

Dressings (regular, reduced-fat, or nonfat)
Blue cheese
Caesar
French
Italian

Mayonnaise
Mayonnaise-type salad dressing
Ranch
Russian
Thousand Island
Vinegar and oil
> Reminder: If you choose regular salad dressing, the serving size is 1 tablespoon; if you choose reduced fat or non-fat, the serving size is 2 tablespoons.

Nuts and Seeds (in the shell)
*Almonds
*Brazil nuts
*Peanuts
*Pecans
*Pistachios
*Sunflower seeds
*Walnuts

OTHER HEALTHY CHOICES

Beverages
Club soda
Coffee
Diet sodas
Fruit beverages, sugar-free
Lemonade, sugar-free
Tea, herbal
Tea, regular
Water

Fast-Food Selections
Caesar salad, regular or side
Chicken Caesar salad
Garden salad
Grilled chicken salad
Grilled chicken sandwich

Meal Replacements
Bars (140 calories or less)
Beverages (230 calories or less when mixed with fat-free milk)

Soups
*Beef bouillon or broth
*Chicken bouillon or broth
*Chicken noodle
*Chicken rice
*Minestrone
*Onion
*Tomato (made with water)
*Tomato vegetable
*Vegetable beef
*Vegetarian vegetable

FOODS TO LIMIT OR AVOID: LOW-RESPONSE COST, LOW-YIELD FOODS

Baked Goods, Breads, Desserts, and Related
Biscuits
Breadsticks
Brownies
Cakes
Coffee cakes
Cookies
Crisps, cobblers, grunts, and slumps
Croissants
Danish pastry
Doughnuts
English muffins (white flour)
Fruitcake
Pancakes
Pies
Rolls and buns (white flour)
Taco shells and fried tortillas
Toaster pastries
Waffles
White bread

Beverages
Alcoholic
    Beer
    Hard liquor

Liqueurs
Wine
Carbonated
All sugar-sweetened soft drinks
Fruit drinks and punches, sugar-sweetened

Dairy Foods
Cheese, full-fat
Blue
Brick
Brie
Camembert
Cheddar
Cream cheese
Gorgonzola
Gouda
Monterey jack
Mozzarella
Meunster
Parmesan
Provolone
Ricotta, whole milk
Romano
Swiss
Cottage Cheese, full-fat (4%)
Cream
Half-and-half
Heavy whipping cream
Light, coffee, or table
Light whipping cream
Sour cream
Whipped cream
Cream, imitation
Coffee whitener
Dessert topping
Desserts
Custard
Frozen dessert bars
Ice cream, full-fat

      Ice cream, soft serve
      Pudding
      Yogurt, frozen
      Yogurt, full-fat, sweetened
Dips
Eggs (cooked in butter or margarine)
Milk and milk products
      Chocolate milk
      Eggnog
      Evaporated, whole
      Malted milk
      Milk shakes
      Sweetened condensed milk
      Whole milk

Fats and Oils
Butter
Margarine
Vegetable shortening

Fast Foods
Bacon cheeseburger
Breakfast sandwich on biscuit or muffin
Burritos, all varieties
Cheeseburger
Croissant sandwich
Double cheeseburger or hamburger
Fish fillet sandwich
Fish sandwich
French fries
Fried chicken (pieces)
Fried chicken sandwich
Ham and cheese sandwich
Hamburger
Hot dog
Onion rings
Pizza
Roast beef sandwich

Submarine sandwich (hero, hoagie, grinder, po' boy, wedge)
Tacos
Turkey club sandwich

Fish and Shellfish
Fried fish
Fried fish and shellfish products, (e.g., fish sticks and popcorn
    shrimp)

Fruits, canned or frozen, in heavy syrup or sweetened
Applesauce
Apricots
Blackberries
Blueberries
Fruit cocktail
Peaches
Pears
Pineapple
Plums
Prunes
Raspberries
Strawberries

Fruit Juices, sugar-sweetened
Apple
Cranberry juice cocktail
Grape
Grapefruit
Orange
Pineapple
Prune

Grain Products
Pasta and noodles from white flour
White rice

Gravies
Any variety, canned or from a mix

Meats
Beef, high-fat cuts
    Chuck blade
    Ground
    Prime rib
    Rib and ribeye steaks
Lunch meats, full-fat
    Bologna
    Bratwurst
    Brown-and-serve sausage
    Corned beef
    Ham
    Hot dogs
    Kielbasa
    Knockwurst
    Olive loaf
    Pepperoni
    Polish sausage
    Smoked sausage, any kind
    Vienna sausage
Pork
    Bacon, "Canadian"
    Bacon, regular
    Ribs, regular and country
    Sausage
Variety meats
    Brains
    Heart
    Liver
    Sweetbreads
    Tongue
Veal
    Breast
    Cutlets, breaded and fried

Mixed Dishes
Microwaveable dinners and entrees, all varieties

Nuts and Seeds (shelled)
Almonds, dry roasted or oiled, salted, flavored
Cashews, dry roasted or oiled, salted
Mixed nuts, all varities
Peanuts, all varieties
Pecans
Sunflower seeds
Trail mix
Walnuts

Poultry
Chicken patty, breaded and fried
Fried chicken
Turkey and gravy, frozen
Turkey patty, breaded and fried

Snack Foods
Bagel chips
Cheese curls
Cheese puffs
Corn chips
Crackers
Popcorn, popped with oil (microwave or stovetop)
Potato chips
Potato sticks
Pretzels
Tortilla chips

Soups
Any cream-style soup

Sweets and Sweeteners
Apple butter
Butterscotch topping
Caramel topping
Candy, all varieties
Chocolate, all varieties
Fruit roll-ups

Fudge topping
Gelatin desserts, sugar-sweetened
Honey
Jams and jellies, sugar-sweetened
Marshmallows
Marshmallow topping
Popsicles
Sugar, all varieties
Syrups, all varieties

Vegetables, regular and starchy
Corn, cream-style
Potatoes
    Au gratin
    French fried
    Hash brown
    Home-fried
    Mashed
    Potato puffs
    Scalloped
Spinach
    Creamed
    Soufflé
Sweet potatoes
    Candied
    Canned
Vegetables, any kind, canned or frozen in sauce

Appendix C

Workout Diary

Use this diary to keep track of your exercise performance. Recording your progress in this manner is essential for building self-confidence and self-efficacy (your level of competence and mastery), increasing your motivation, and integrating exercise into your lifestyle. The sample entry provides an example of how to record your exercise activities and performance.

DAY OF THE WEEK	TIME	ACTIVITY	DURATION/LEVEL OF EFFORT
Sample	7 am	Walking	30 minutes, 2 miles
	5 pm	Weight training routine	Leg extensions: 30 lbs, 12 repetitions; 40 lbs, 10 repetitions
			Leg curls: 40 lbs, 9 repetitions; 45 lbs, 8 repetitions
			Sit-ups: 25 repetitions
			Bench press: 10 lbs, 12 repetitions; 15 lbs, 8 repetitions
			Shoulder press: 10 lbs, 12 repetitions; 15 lbs, 10 repetitions
			Arm curls: 10 lbs, 12 repetitions; 15 lbs, 8 repetitions
Sunday			

(continued on next page)

DAY OF THE WEEK	TIME	ACTIVITY	DURATION/LEVEL OF EFFORT
Monday			
Tuesday			
Wednesday			
Thursday			
Friday			
Saturday			

Appendix D

Bibliography

PART ONE: UNLOCKING THE DOORS TO PERMANENT WEIGHT LOSS

Associated Press. 2002. Fast food pops up at nation's top hospitals. Wire service report, June 16.

Bellisle, F. 1999. Food choice, appetite and physical activity. *Public Health Nutrition* 2: 357–361.

Birch, L.L. 1992. Children's preferences for high-fat foods. *Nutrition Reviews* 50: 249–255.

Center for Science in the Public Interest (CSPI). 2000. Sugar intake hit all-time high in 1999. CSPI Press release, May 18.

Drewnowski, A. 1995. Energy intake and sensory properties of food. *The American Journal of Clinical Nutrition* 62: 1081S–1085S.

Editor. 2001. Intervening in the obesity epidemic. *Patient Care*, August 15, pp. 92–107.

French, S.A., et al. 2001. Environmental influences on eating and physical activity. *Annual Review of Public Health* 22: 309–335.

Gleick, E. 1999. Get thin quick—an update. Time.com, October 25.

Hamilton, M.A., et al. 2000. The life stages of weight: setting achievable goals appropriate to each woman. *International Journal of Fertility* 45: 5–12.

Hansen, B.C. 2001. Emerging strategies for weight management. *Postgraduate Medicine Special Report* June: 3–9.

Harris, M.B., et al. 1990. Feeling fat: motivations, knowledge, and attitudes. *Psychological Reports* 67: 1191–1202.

Manore, M.M. 1996. Chronic dieting in active women: what are the health consequences? *Women's Health Issues* 6: 332–341.

Nestle, M., et al. 2000. Halting the obesity epidemic: a public health poll. *Public Health Reports* 115: 12–24.

Roberts, P. 1998. The new food anxiety. *Psychology Today*, March–April. Online.

Turner, S.L., et al. 1997. The influence of fashion magazines on the body image satisfaction of college women: an exploratory analysis. *Adolescence* 32: 603–614.

Young, L.R., et al. 2002. The contribution of expanding portion sizes to the U.S. obesity epidemic. *Research and Practice* 92: 246–249.

PART TWO: THE SEVEN KEYS TO PERMANENT WEIGHT LOSS

CHAPTER 4: Key One—Right Thinking

Nir, Z., et al. 1995. Relationship among self-esteem, internal-external locus of control, and weight change after participation in a weight reduction program. *Journal of Clinical Psychology* 51: 482–490.

Saltzer, E.B. 1982. The weight locus of control scale: a specific measure for obesity research. *Journal of Personality Assessment* 46: 620–628.

CHAPTER 5: Key Two—Healing Feelings

Puhl, R., et al. 2001. Bias, discrimination, and obesity. *Obesity Research* 9: 788–805.

CHAPTER 6: Key Three—A No-Fail Environment

American Cancer Society. 2002. Cancer facts & figures.

American Lung Association. 2002. Trends in tobacco use.

French, S.A., et al. 2001. Environmental influences on eating and physical activity. *Annual Review of Public Health* 22: 309–335.

Goldfield, G.S., et al. 2002. Can fruits and vegetables and activities substitute for snack foods? *Health Psychology* 21: 299–303.

Nestle, M., et al. 1998. Behavioral and social influences on food choice. *Nutrition Reviews* 56: S50–64.

Poston, W.S., et al. 1999. Obesity is an environmental issue. *Atherosclerosis* 146: 201–209.

Robins, L.N., et al. 1975. Narcotic use in southeast Asia and afterward. An interview study of 898 Vietnam returnees. *Archives of General Psychiatry* 32: 955–961.

Rodin, J., et al. 1975. Causes and consequences of time perception differences in overweight and normal weight people. *Journal of Personality and Social Psychology* 31: 898–904.

Rodin, J. 1985. Insulin levels, hunger, and food intake: an example of feedback loops in body weight reduction. *Health Psychology* 4: 1–24.

Schachter, S. 1968. Obesity and eating. *Science* 161: 751:756.

CHAPTER 7: Key Four—Mastery Over Food and Impulse Eating

Adams, S.O., et al. 1986. Weight loss: a comparison of group and individual interventions. *Journal of the American Dietetic Association* 86: 485–490.

DeLucia-Waack, J.L. 1999. Supervision for counselors working with eating disorders groups; countertransference issues related to body image, food, and weight. *Journal of Counseling and Development* 77:379–388.

Foreyt, J.P., et al. 1993. Evidence for success of behavioral modification in weight loss and control. *Annals of Internal Medicine* 119: 698–701.

French, S.A., et al. 2001. Environmental influences on eating and physical activity. *Annual Review of Public Health* 22: 309–335.

French, S.A., et al. 2000. Fast food restaurant use among women in the Pound of Prevention study: dietary, behavioral and demographic correlates. *International Journal of Obesity* 24: 1353–1359.

Guertin, T. 1999. Eating behavior of bulimics, self-identified binge eaters, and non-eating-disordered individuals: what differentiates these populations? *Clinical Psychology Review* 19: 1–25.

Keller, C., et al. 1997. Strategies for weight control success in adults. *The Nurse Practitioner* 22: 33, 37–38.

Lasure, L.C., et al. 1996. Biblical behavior modification. *Behavior Research and Therapy* 34: 563–566.

McCartney, J. 1995. Addictive behaviors: Relationship factors and their perceived influence on change. *Genetic, Social and General Psychology Monographs* 121: 41, ff.

Pearcy, S.M., et al. 2002. Food intake and meal patterns of weight-stable and weight-gaining persons. *American Journal of Clinical Nutrition* 76: 107–112.

Stunkard, A., et al. 2003. Two forms of disordered eating in obesity: binge eating and night eating. *International Journal of Obesity* 27: 1–12.

CHAPTER 8: Key Five—High-Response Cost, High-Yield Nutrition

Brand-Miller, J.C., et al. 2002. Glycemic index and obesity. *The American Journal of Clinical Nutrition* 76: 281S–285S.

Foreyt, J.P., et al. 1986. Soup consumption as a behavioral weight loss strategy. *Journal of the American Dietetic Association* 86: 524–526.

Gamel, K. 2002. Study links high-carbs to cancer. Associated Press wire report, May 3.

Jordan, H.A., et al. 1981. Role of food characteristics in behavioral change and weight loss. *Journal of the American Dietetic Association* 99: 24–29.

Kleiner, S.M. 1999. Water: an essential but overlooked ingredient. *Journal of the American Dietetic Association* 99: 200–206.

Ludwig, D.S. 2000. Dietary glycemic index and obesity. *Journal of Nutrition* 130: 280S–283S.

———. 2002. The glycemic index. *Journal of the American Medical Association* 287: 2414–2423.

Roberts, S.B., et al. 2002. The influence of dietary composition on energy intake and body weight. *Journal of the American College of Nutrition* 21: 140S–145S.

Rolls, B.J., et al. 1990. Foods with different satiating effects in humans. *Appetite* 15: 115–126.

CHAPTER 9: Key Six—Intentional Exercise

Racette, S.B., et al. 1995. Exercise enhances dietary compliance during moderate energy restriction in obese women. *The American Journal of Clinical Nutrition* 62: 345–349.

Saelens, B.E., et al. 1999. The rate of sedentary activities determines the reinforcing value of physical activity. *Health Psychology* 18: 655–659.

Scully, D., et al. 1998. Physical exercise and psychological well being: a critical review. *British Journal of Sports Medicine* 32: 111–120.

Sherwood, N.E., et al. 2000. The behavioral determinants of exercise: implications for physical activity interventions. *Annual Review of Nutrition* 20: 21–44.

CHAPTER 10: Key Seven—Your Circle of Support

Patel, K.A., et al. 2001. Impact of moods and social context on eating behavior. *Appetite* 36: 111–118.

PART THREE: POWERFUL INSIGHTS

CHAPTER 11: When You Can't Lose Weight: Are You Weight Loss Resistant?

Anderson, J.W., et al. 1995. Meta-analysis of effects of soy protein intake on serum lipids. *New England Journal of Medicine* 333: 276–282.

Cohen, N., et al. 1995. Oral vanadyl sulfate improves hepatic and peripheral insulin sensitivity in patients with non-insulin-dependent diabetes mellitus. *The Journal of Clinical Investigation* 95: 2501–2509.

Cunningham, J.J. 1998. Micronutrients as nutriceutical interventions in diabetes mellitus. *Journal of the American College of Nutrition* 17: 7–10.

Dulloo, A.G., et al. 1999. Efficacy of a green tea extract rich in catechin polyphenols and caffeine and increasing 24-h energy expenditure and fat oxidation in humans. *American Journal of Clinical Nutrition* 70: 1040–1050.

————. 2000. Green tea and thermogenesis: interactions between catechinpolyphenols, caffeine and sympathetic activity. *International Journal of Obesity* 24: 252–258.

Feller, A.G., et al. 1988. Role of carnitine in human nutrition. *Journal of Nutrition* 118: 541–547.

Han, L.K., et al. 1999. Anti-obesity action of oolong tea. *International Journal of Obesity* 23: 98–105.

Harland, B.F., et al. 1994. Is vanadium of human nutritional importance yet? *Journal of the American Dietetic Association* 94: 891–894.

John, R., et al. 1999. A randomized trial comparing the effect of casein with that of soy protein containing varying amounts of isoflavones on plasma concentrations of lipids and lipoproteins. *Archives of Internal Medicine* 159: 2070.

Kanter, M.M., et al. 1995. Antioxidants, carnitine, and choline as putative ergogenic aids. *International Journal of Sports Nutrition* 5: S120–131.

Kendler, B.S., et al. 1986. Carnitine: an overview of its role in preventive medicine. *Preventive Medicine* 15: 373–390.

Minchoff, L.E., et al. 1996. Recognition and management of this metabolic disorder in primary care. (Syndrome X). *The Nurse Practitioner* 21: 74–80.

Nielson F. 1999. Requirements for vanadium and impact on human health. Food and Nutrition Board Forum presented at Annual Meeting of the Federation of American Societies for Experimental Biology, April, 17–21, Washington, DC.

Otto, R.M., et al. 1987. The effect of L-carnitine supplementation on endurance exercise. *Medicine and Science in Sports and Exercise* 19: S68.

Reaven, G.M. 2000. Diet and syndrome X. *Current Atherosclerosis Reports* 2: 503–507.

Rimm, A.A., et al. 1988. A weight shape index for assessing risk of disease. *Journal of Clinical Epidemiology* 41: 459–465.

Roberts, S.B., et al. 2002. The influence of dietary composition on energy intake and body weight. *Journal of the American College of Nutrition* 21: 140S–145S.

Singh, R.B., et al. 1999. Effect of hydrosoluble coenzyme Q10 on blood pressures and insulin resistance in hypertensive patients with coronary artery disease. *Journal of Human Hypertension* 13: 203–208.

Singh, R.B., et al. 1999. Serum concentration of lipoprotein (a) decreases on treatment with hydrosoluble coenzyme Q10 in patients with coronary artery disease: discovery of a new role. *International Journal of Cardiology* 68: 23–29.

Weber, C., et al. 1994. Antioxidative effect of dietary coenzyme Q10 in human blood plasma. *International Journal for Vitamin and Nutrition Research* 64: 311–315.

Willard, M.D. 1991. Obesity: types and treatment. *American Family Physician* 43: 2099–2108.

Index

About the Author

Phillip C. McGraw, Ph.D. is the #1 *New York Times* bestselling author of *Life Strategies*, *Relationship Rescue*, and *Self Matters*. He is the host of the nationally syndicated, daily one-hour series *Dr. Phil*. One of the world's foremost experts in the field of human functioning, Dr. McGraw is the cofounder of Courtroom Sciences, Inc., the world's leading litigation consulting firm. Dr. McGraw currently lives in Los Angeles, California, with his wife and two sons.